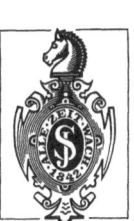

C. Y. Genton

Histopathology of the Female Genital Tract

With 157 Figures

Springer-Verlag
Berlin Heidelberg New York Tokyo 1983

Priv.-Doz. Dr. CLAUDE YVES GENTON
Institut für Pathologie der Universität Zürich,
Schmelzbergstraße 12, CH-8091 Zürich

ISBN 978-3-540-12512-9   ISBN 978-3-642-50256-9 (eBook)
DOI 10.1007/978-3-642-50256-9

Library of Congress Cataloging in Publication Data
Genton, C. Y. (Claude Yves), 1940–
  Histopathology of the female genital tract.

  Bibliography: p.
  Includes index.
  1. Pathology, Gynecological. 2. Histology, Patho-
logical. I. Title. [DNLM 1. Genital diseases, female
–Pathology. 2. Genital neoplasms, Female–Pathology.
WP 140 G338h]
RG77.G46 1983   618.1′07   83-10521

The use of registered names, trademarks, etc. in this publication does not im-
ply, even in the absence of a specific statement, that such names are exempt
from the relevant protective laws and regulations and therefore free for gen-
eral use.

Product Liability: The publisher can give no guarantee for information about
drug dosage and application thereof contained in this book. In every individual case the respective user must check its accuracy by consulting other
pharmaceutical literature.

2123/3130-543210

Contents

I. Histopathology of the Vulva

References

Boehm F, Morris JMcL (1971) Paget's disease and apocrine gland carcinoma of the vulva. Obstet Gynecol 38:185–192

Chamlian DL, Taylor HB (1972) Primary carcinoma of Bartholin's gland. A report of 24 patients. Obstet Gynecol 39:489–494

Charles AH (1972) Carcinoma of the vulva. Br Med J I:397–402

DiSaia PJ, Rutledge F, Smith JP (1971) Sarcoma of the vulva. Report of 12 patients. Obstet Gynecol 38:180–184

Hilliard GD, Massey FM, O'Toole RV (1979) Vulvar neoplasia in the young. Am J Obstet Gynecol 135:185–188

Iversen T, Aalders GJ, Christensen A et al. (1980) Squamous cell carcinoma of the vulva: a review of 424 patients, 1956–1974. Gynecol Oncol 9:271–279

Wade TR, Kopf AW, Ackermann AB (1979) Bowenoid papulosis of the genitalia. Arch Dermatol 115:306–308

Fig. 1. Lichen sclerosus et atrophicus. This lesion of the vulva appears clinically as a leukoplakia with or without induration. Histologically, there is hyperkeratosis and atrophy of the squamous epithelium, edema, and homogenization of the collagen in the upper dermis as well as an inflammatory infiltrate in the middermis. × 85

Fig. 2. Bartholin's gland. The main ducts of this tubuloalveolar gland are lined with transitional epithelium. The gland acini are composed of simple mucus-secreting cells. A focal squamous metaplasia may be occasionally observed. × 135

Fig. 3. Chronic Bartholinitis. The transitional epithelium is partly exfoliated and may be absent. The stroma is severely infiltrated with lymphocytes and plasmocytes. × 210

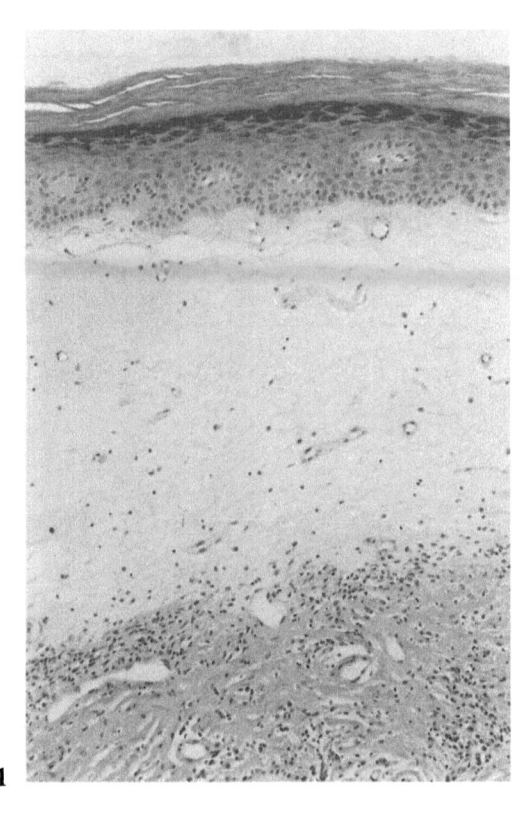

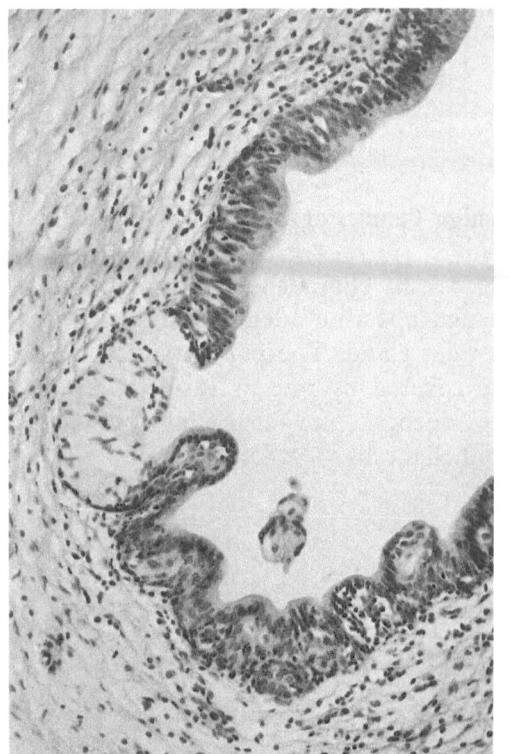

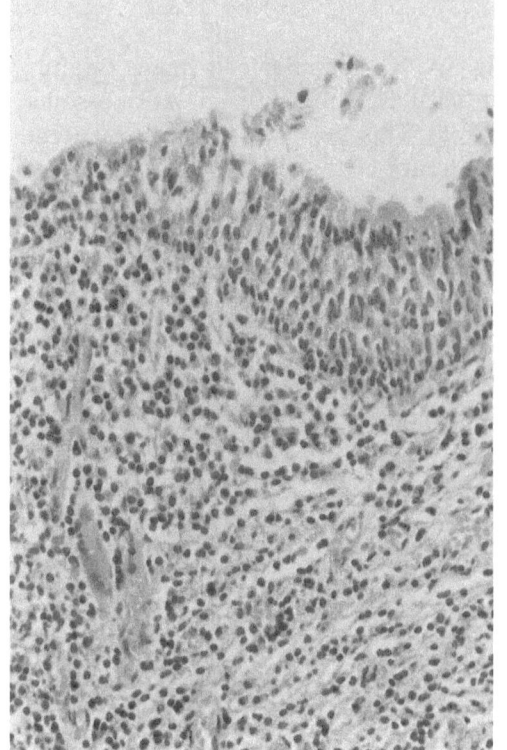

1

2

3

Benign Tumors of the Vulva

Fig. 4 A, B. Hidradenoma   papilliferum. Benign apocrine adenoma arising from a sweat gland. The papillary structures are covered by one or two cell layers, the deepest one consisting of myo-epithelial cells. *A* ×85; *B* ×335

Fig. 5 A, B. Granular cell tumor (granular cell myoblastoma, Abrikossoff's tumor). This tumor is not encapsulated. The tumor cells are large and polygonal. Their cytoplasm is abundant, pale, and contains numerous eosinophilic PAS-positive granules. The cell borders are indistinct. The centrally located nuclei are small, round to oval, and hyperchromatic. Some multinucleated cells may be present. *A* ×135; *B* ×210

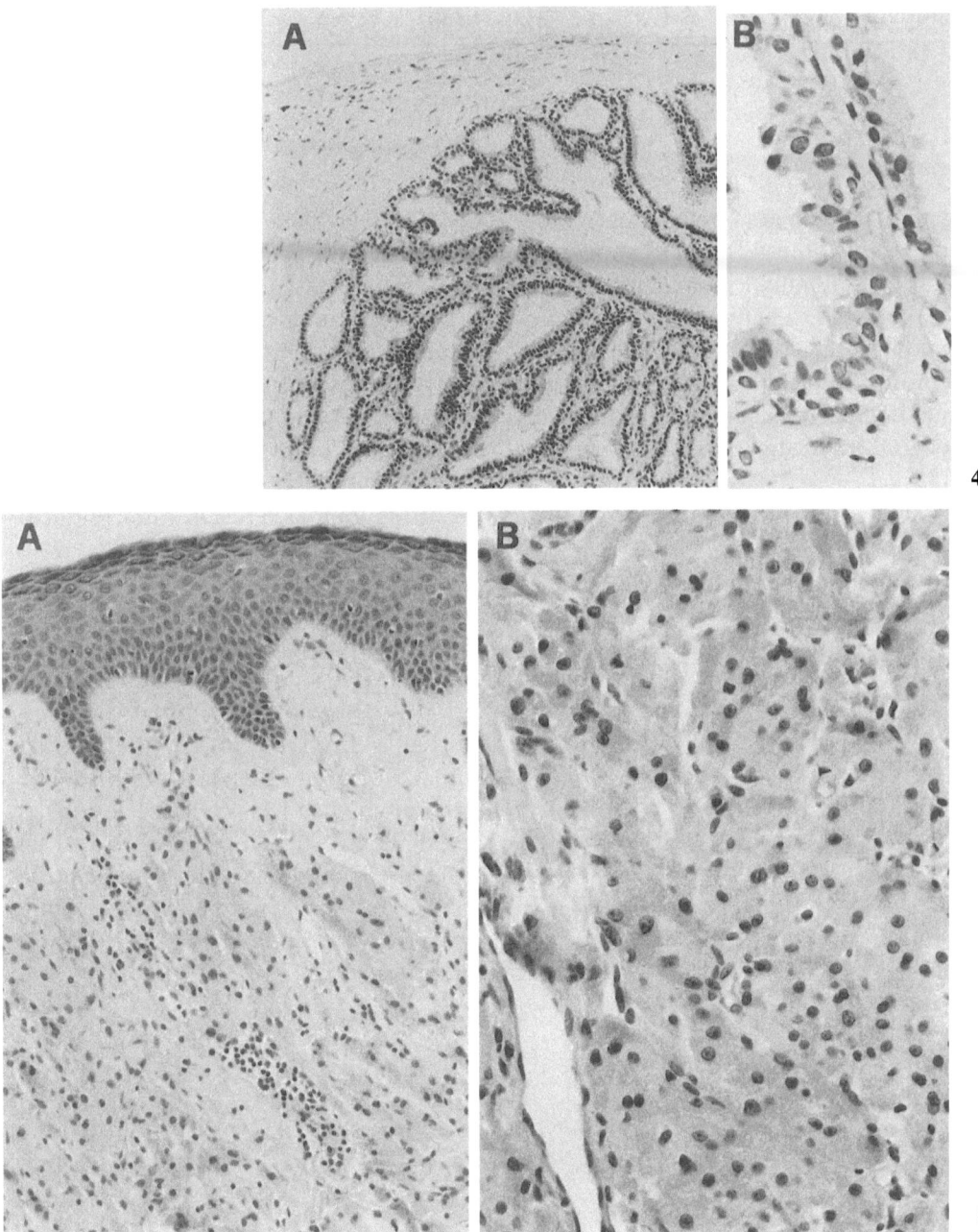

4

5

5

Fig. 6. Condylomata acuminata. Morphologically, these lesions appear as acanthopapillomas with or without hyperkeratosis. There are no pathognomonic histologic criteria for the specific diagnosis of these viral lesions, although some degree of koilocytosis and lymphocytic infiltration is often present. × 135

Fig. 7. Condyloma acuminata after treatment with podophyllin. Podophyllin may be used as a therapeutic agent in the local treatment of condylomata acuminata. This substance acts upon the G2 phase of the cell cycle and causes mitotic arrest in the metaphase. This cytotoxic action may lead to dysplastic epithelial changes, which can persist as long as 6 weeks after application. × 135

Fig. 8. Bowenoid papulosis (23-year-old patient). This probably viral-induced lesion is histologically often indistinguishable from an intraepithelial carcinoma or from Bowen's disease. The differential diagnosis of these lesions is based upon clinical data alone. This pigmented and usually multicentric disease affects predominantly young women. The optimal therapy is still under discussion. × 135

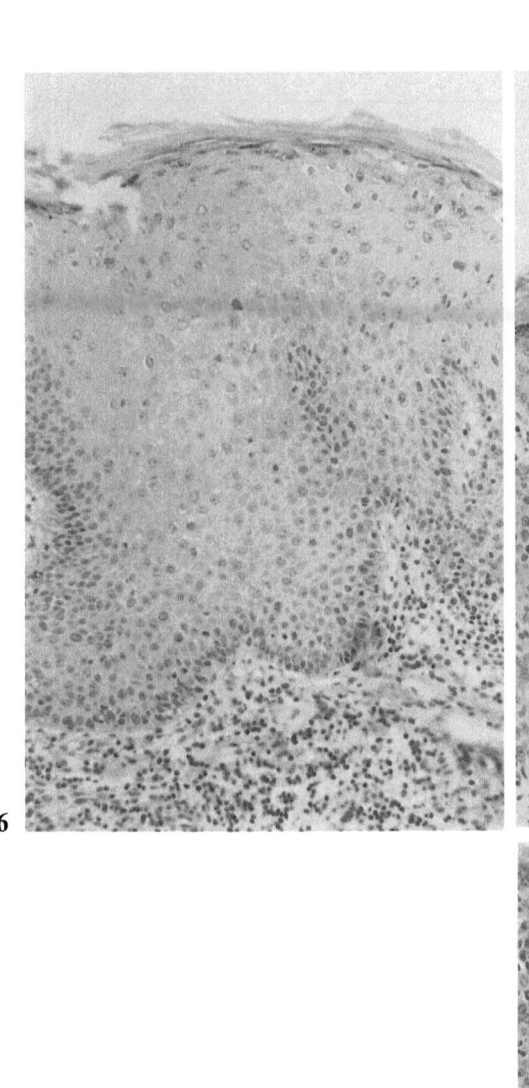

6

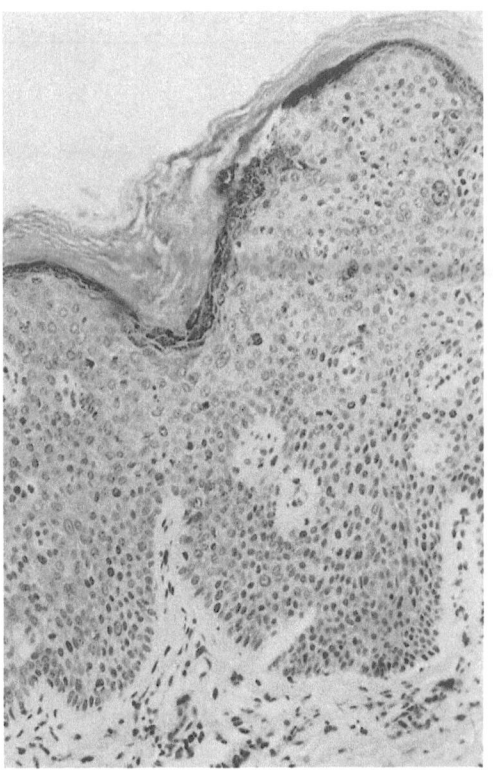

7

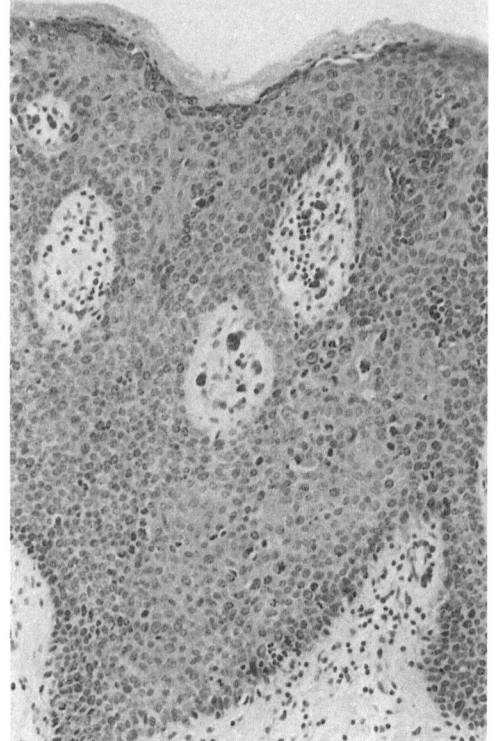

8

Fig. 9. Intraepithelial carcinoma (carcinoma in situ). In this lesion, cellular and nuclear atypia is present in all layers of the squamous epithelium, although some degree of stratification may persist. × 135

Fig. 10. Paget's disease. The so-called Paget's cells are found predominantly in the basal and parabasal cell layers of the squamous epithelium. These cells are large and round or oval. The nuclei are vesicular and basophilic. The cytoplasm is abundant, pale, and vacuolated. It contains various mucopolysaccharides, which are PAS-positive. In contrast to Paget's disease of the nipple, in which an underlying ductal carcinoma is practically always present, a subjacent adenocarcinoma is found in only 25%–40% of vulvar Paget's disease. This last lesion represents most often a multicentric primary intraepithelial carcinoma. × 335

Fig. 11 A, B. Bowen's disease. This lesion represents a particular form of intraepithelial carcinoma which may become invasive after many years. The squamous epithelium is acanthotic, often hyperkeratotic, and its stratification is severely disturbed. Mitoses occur in all cell layers (A × 105). **B**: so-called clumping cells, multinucleated cells, as well as individual cell keratinization are further typical characteristics of this lesion. × 335

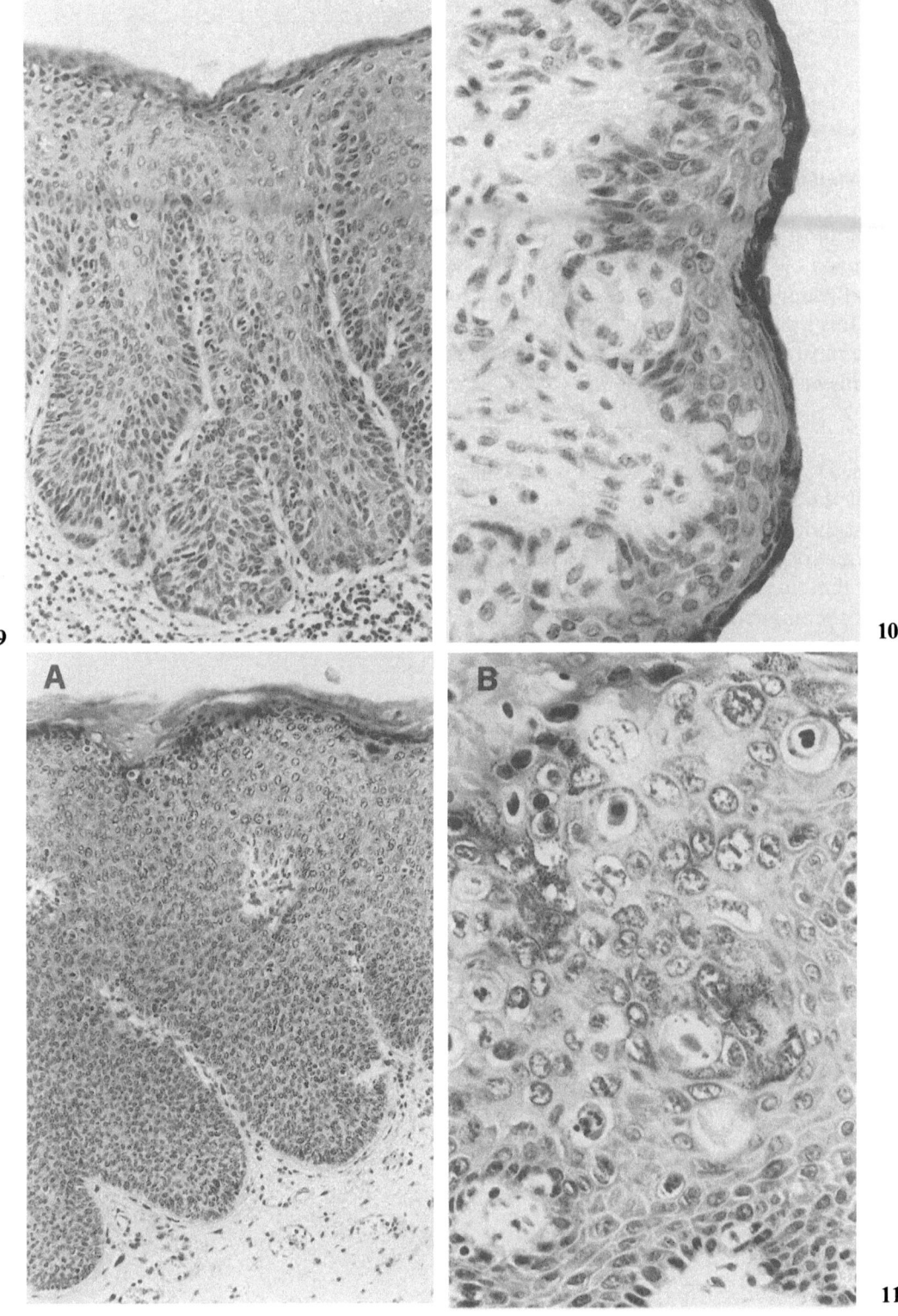

9

Malignant Tumors of the Vulva

The most common primary malignant tumor of the vulva is the squamous cell carcinoma, which is often well differentiated. It occurs mostly in elderly women. Malignant melanoma, adenocarcinoma, and sarcoma are very rare forms of cancer in this location. Metastatic tumors occasionally involve the vulva. Cervical cancer is the most frequent primary lesion, followed by carcinoma of the endometrium and kidney and choriocarcinoma.

Fig. 12. Well-differentiated squamous cell carcinoma. Tongues of neoplastic squamous epithelium with keratin-pearl formation invade the stroma. The nuclei of the tumor cells most often exhibit very prominent nucleoli. ×85

Fig. 13. Poorly differentiated squamous cell carcinoma. The solid tumor tissue consists of polymorphic epithelial cells with numerous mitotic figures. Keratin formation is absent. ×210

Fig. 14. Adenocarcinoma. One of the rarest primary vulvar malignancies, which develops from Bartholin's gland or from some other mucus-secreting gland of the introitus area. ×210

Fig. 15. Fibrosarcoma. The tumor tissue is undifferentiated and consists of spindle-shaped cells. Mitotic figures are numerous. The tumor cells have polymorphic nuclei and poorly developed cytoplasm. ×335

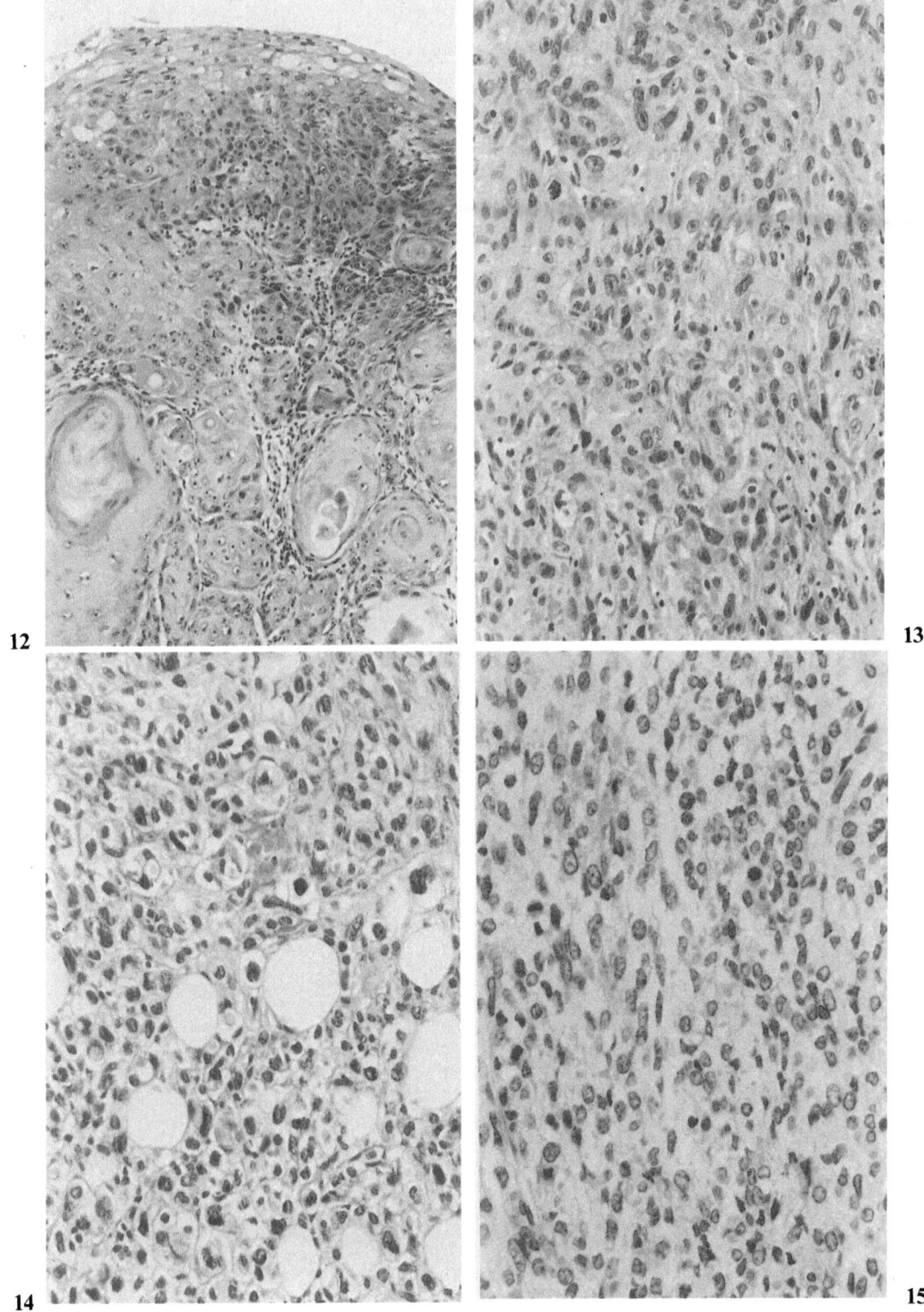

12   13

14   15

II. Histopathology of the Vagina

References

Bibbo M, Gill WB, Azizi F et al. (1977) Follow-up study of male and female offspring of DES-exposed mothers. Obstet Gynecol 49:1–8

Davos I, Abell MR (1976) Sarcomas of the vagina. Obstet Gynecol 47:342–350

Perez CA, Arneson AN, Galaktos A et al. (1973) Malignant tumors of the vagina. Cancer 31:36–44

Robboy SJ, Scully RE, Welch WR et al. (1977) Intrauterine diethylstilbestrol exposure and its consequences. Arch Pathol Lab Med 101:1–5

Fig. 16. Normal mucosa of the adult vagina. The luminal surface is lined with nonkeratinizing squamous epithelium, which exhibits under estrogenic stimulation quite prominent superficial cell layers that contain glycogen. Some degree of parakeratosis may be present. ×210

Fig. 17. Normal mucosa of the infant vagina. The squamous epithelium is very thin and consists only of a few cell layers. In the stroma lie thin-walled blood vessels. ×210

Fig. 18. Normal vaginal mucosa after menopause. The squamous epithelium is thin and consists predominantly of parabasal cells. No glycogen is present and the mucosa does not stain with an iodine solution (Schiller's test). ×210

Fig. 19. Vaginal adenosis. The luminal surface is focally lined with mucinous columnar epithelium resembling that of the normal endocervical mucosa. Some degree of squamous metaplasia is usually found. Some mucus-secreting glandular structures may also be present in the lamina propria. ×135

This lesion is most common in the prenatal diethylstilboestrol (DES)-exposed female. Major questions about the relationship between vaginal adenosis and clear-cell carcinoma still remain to be answered.

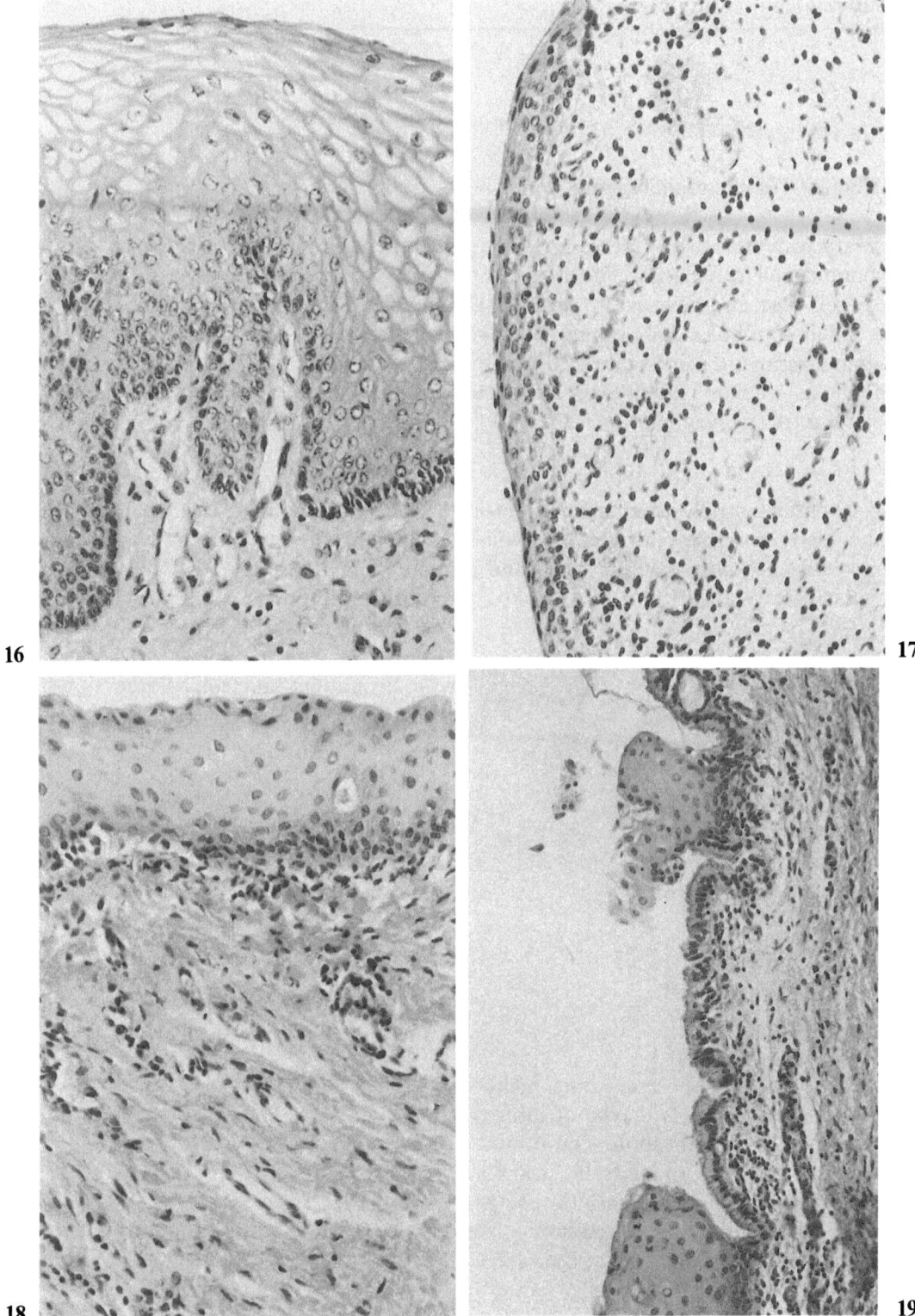

16

17

18

19

Malignant Tumors of the Vagina

Primary carcinoma of the vagina is rarely encountered and is most often a squamous cell carcinoma. The majority of reported adenocarcinomas are of the clear-cell type and develop in prenatal DES-exposed females. Vaginal metastases are much commoner as primary vaginal malignancies. Tumors arising from the endometrium and cervix are the commonest sources of metastases. Choriocarcinoma as well as carcinoma of the ovaries and kidney may also occasionally metastasize to the vagina.

Fig. 20. Endometrial carcinoma metastatic to the vagina. Partly exophytic tumor tissue, which exhibits solid and papillary areas. ×210

Fig. 21. Primary vaginal squamous cell carcinoma. The invading tumor tissue is moderately differentiated. The stroma is severely infiltrated with lymphocytes. The tumor cells are arranged in small groups, they have polymorphic nuclei with prominent nucleoli. Some tumor cells show some degree of keratinization. ×135

Fig. 22A, B. Primary malignant melanoma of the vagina. This type of tumor is very rare in this location. The tumor tissue grows partly in large solid strands **A**, partly in a dissolute fashion **B**. A considerable junctional activity is present in the adjacent squamous epithelium **B**. *A* ×335; *B* ×135

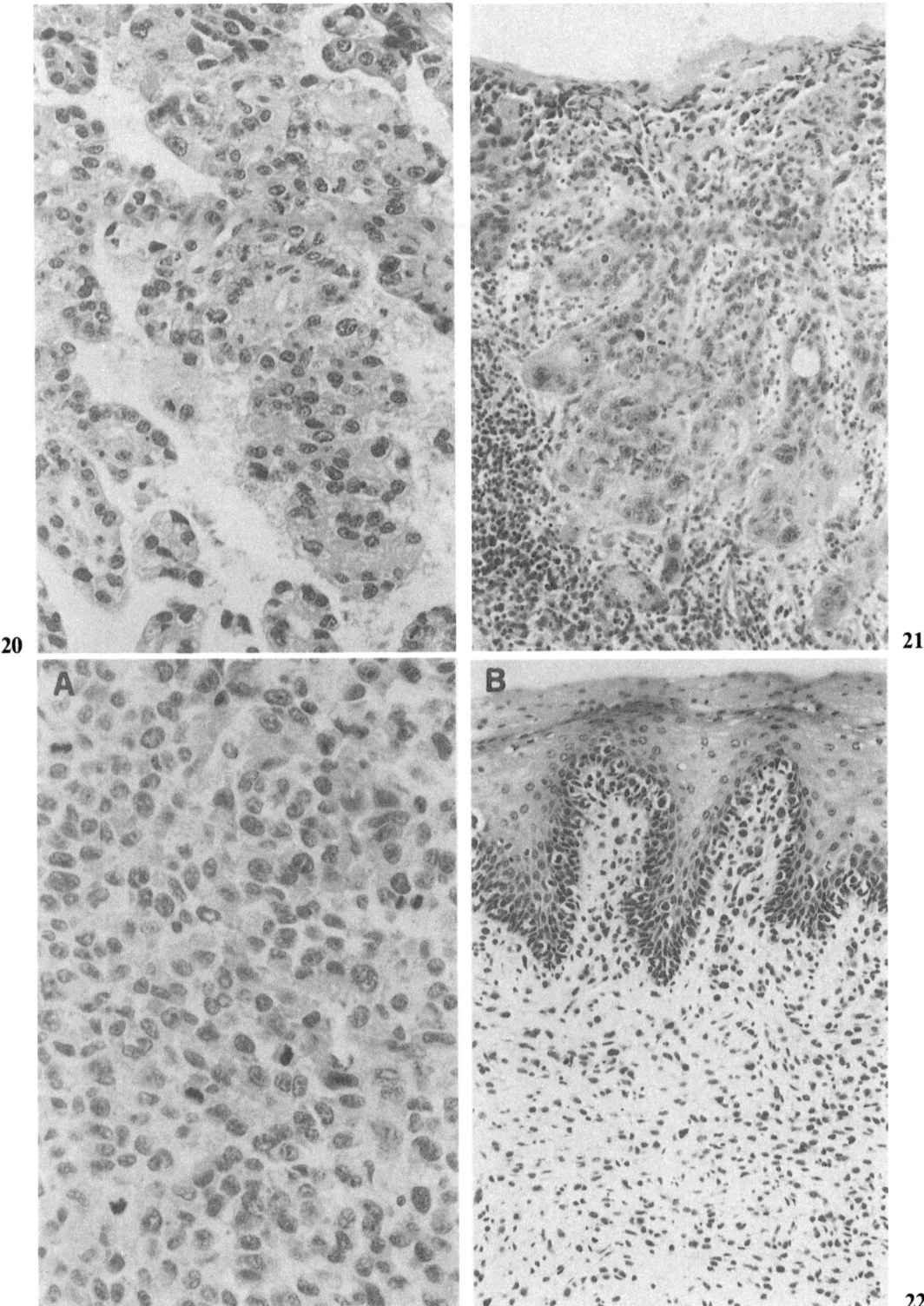

20

21

A

B

22

17

III. Histopathology of the Cervix

References

Burghardt E (1972) Histologische Früh-diagnose des Zervixkrebses. Lehrbuch und Atlas. Thieme, Stuttgart

Genton CY (1974) Adenoid cystic carcinoma of the uterine cervix. Obstet Gynecol 43:905–908

Herbst AL, Robboy SJ, Scully RE et al. (1974) Clear-cell adenocarcinoma of the vagina and cervix in girls: an analysis of 170 registry cases. Am J Obstet Gynecol 119:713–723

Lohe KJ (1978) Early squamous cell carcinoma of the uterine cervix. I. Definition and histology. Gynecol Oncol 6:10–30

Fig. 23. Normal exocervical epithelium. The nonkeratinizing squamous epithelium shows normal maturation with basal, parabasal, intermediate, and superficial cells. The latter contain large amounts of glycogen and stain strongly with iodine solution (Schiller's test). ×210

Fig. 24. Sharp border between normal and abnormal epithelium. The abnormal epithelium on the *right* displays a prominent stratum spinosum, parakeratosis, and a lack of glycogen-containing superficial cells. The various pathologic changes found in the squamous epithelium (dysplastic changes) are always sharply separated from one another, this in contrast to areas with reactive inflammatory "atypia." ×210

Cervical Intraepithelial Neoplasia

Fig. 25. Abnormal exocervical epithelium. In this case, clinically a leukoplakia, the epithelium shows marked hyperkeratosis and a prominent stratum spinosum. ×270

Fig. 26. Mild dysplasia. The parabasal cell layer is thickened due to retarded cell maturation. Some mitoses are present in the lower third of the epithelium. The nuclei of the parabasal and intermediate cells are enlarged. ×335

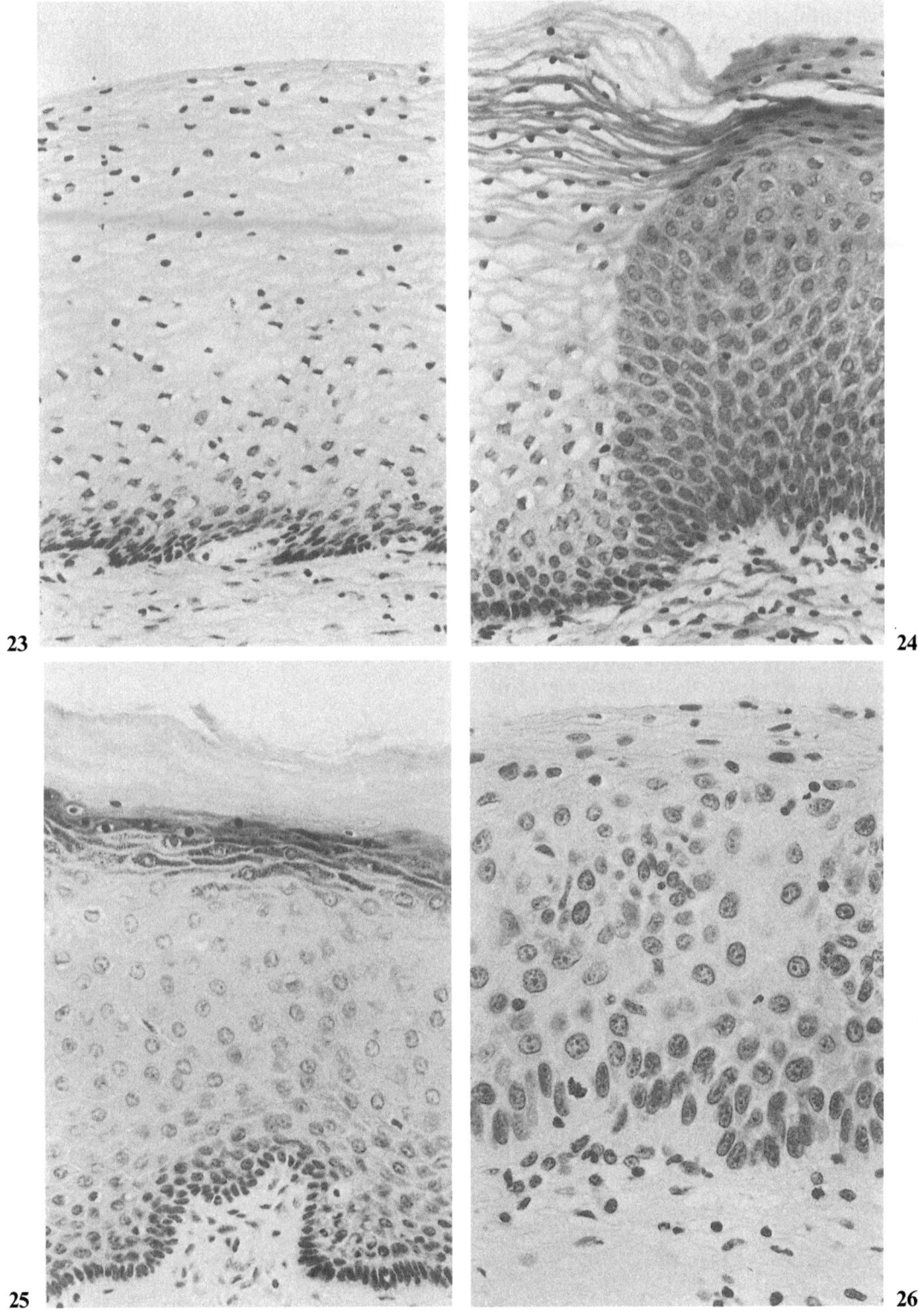

Fig. 27. Moderate dysplasia. The maturation of the squamous cells is retarded and disturbed. The nuclei of the parabasal and intermediate cells are enlarged with a coarse chromatin structure and prominent nucleoli. Mitoses are present in the lower two-thirds of the epithelium. ×270

Fig. 28. Severe dysplasia. Differentiation and maturation of the squamous cells are profoundly disturbed. The nuclei are enlarged in all cell layers, their chromatin structure is coarse, the nucleoli are prominent. Mitoses are present in all cell layers. Only the uppermost cell layers show some degree of maturation and keratinization. ×335

Fig. 29. Carcinoma in situ (CIS). In this condition, a maximum degree of dedifferentiation is found. The cells, however, are often of a greater uniformity as in dysplasias. The nuclei are strongly enlarged, sometimes oval with their long axis perpendicular to the basement membrane. Normal and pathologic mitotic figures are present in all cell layers. ×335

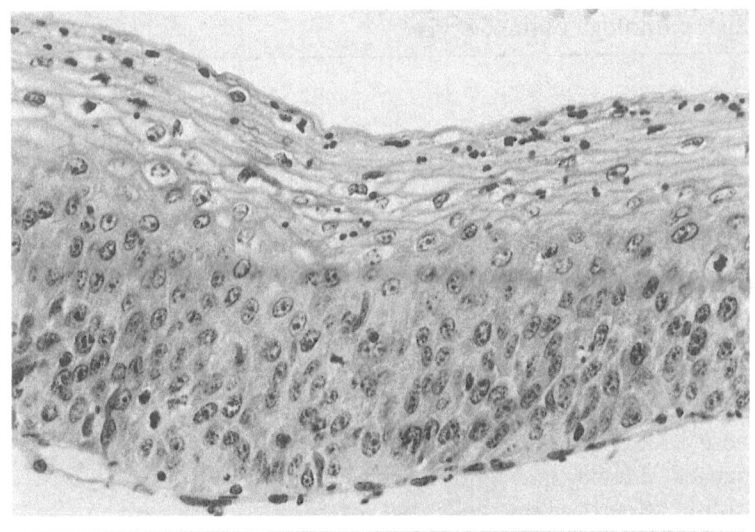

27

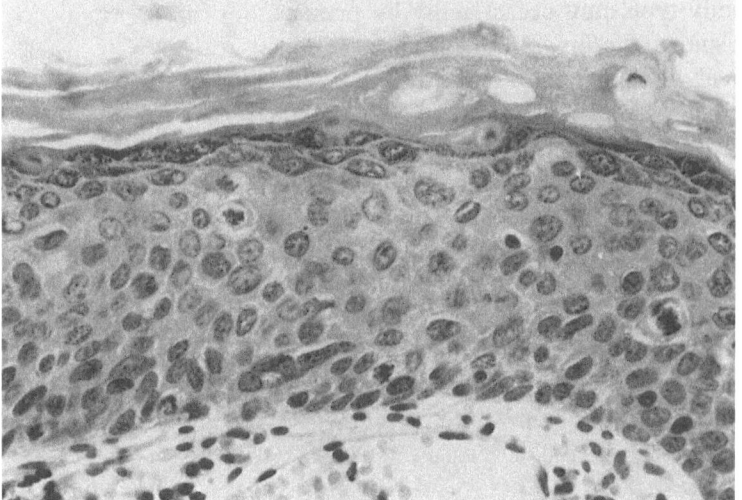

28

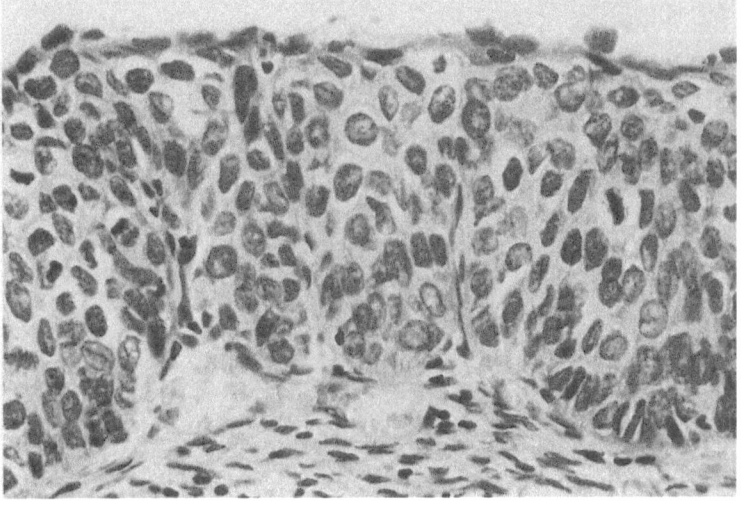

29

Invasive Cervical Neoplasia

Fig. 30. Microinvasive cervical carcinoma. Small tufts of atypical cells break through the basement membrane. In these locations, the stroma shows marked edema and lymphocytic infiltration. Some giant cells of foreign-body type may occasionally be present. Usually, the invading cells show a relatively high degree of maturation. × 210

Fig. 31. Microcarcinoma of the Cervix (stage Ia). This carcinoma is defined as having a maximal depth of infiltration of 5 mm (▷) and a maximal lateral extension of 10 by 10 mm. On the *left* (▶), some cervical glands filled with neoplastic epithelium can be seen (CIS). At this stage, lymph node metastases are found in 1%–2% of cases. × 33

Fig. 32. Invasive front of a microcarcinoma. The stroma is edematous and strongly infiltrated by lymphocytes. The invading tumor cells usually show a moderate degree of maturation. × 135

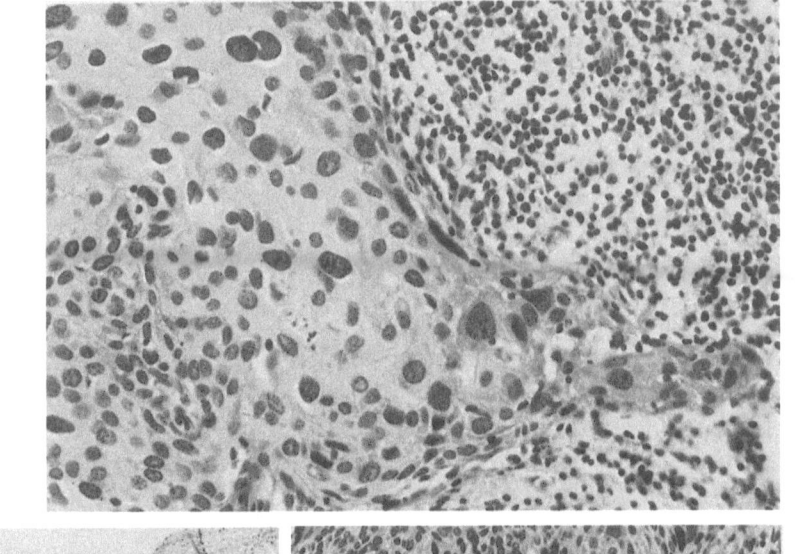

30

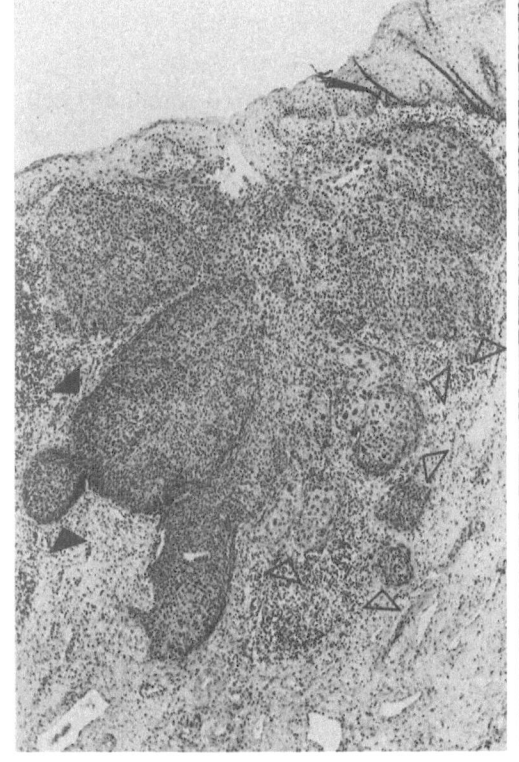

31

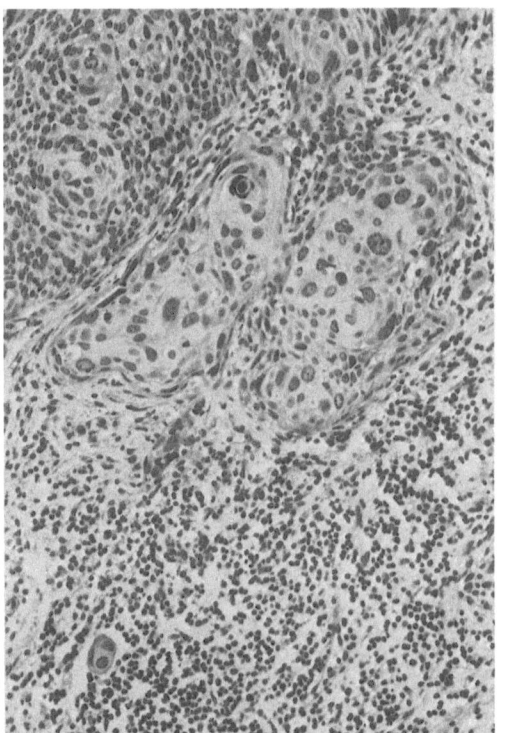

32

The Endocervical Mucosa

Fig. 33. Normal endocervical gland. The glands as well as the surface are lined with monolayered mucinous columnar epithelium. The nuclei are most often basally located. The cytoplasm contains abundant PAS- and alcian-blue-positive mucus. ×335

Fig. 34. Hyperplasia of the reserve cells. A single row of cuboidal reserve cells is seen under the tall columnar endocervical epithelium. These reserve cells may proliferate and form several layers, which will sooner or later develop a squamous cell metaplasia. ×335

Fig. 35. Partly maturated squamous cell metaplasia. The multilayered reserve cells have differentiated into squamous cells and form a distinct stratum spinosum. The endocervical columnar cells may be seen on the epithelium surface. These glandular cells will be exfoliated. ×335

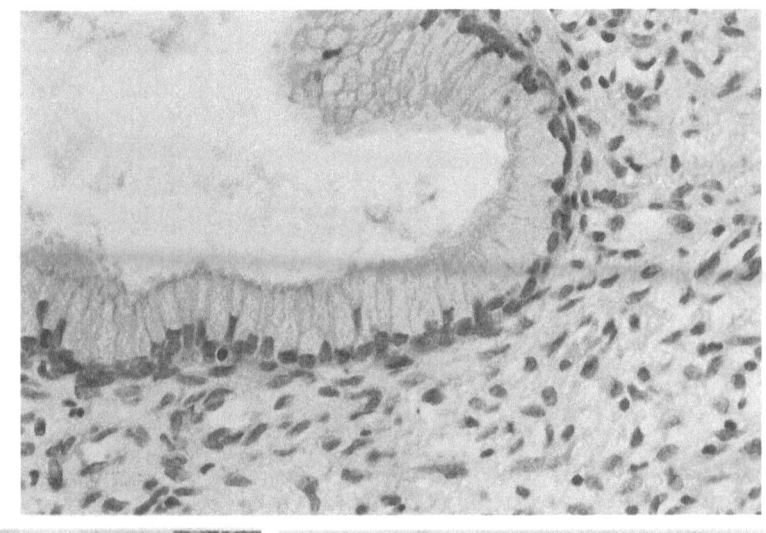

33

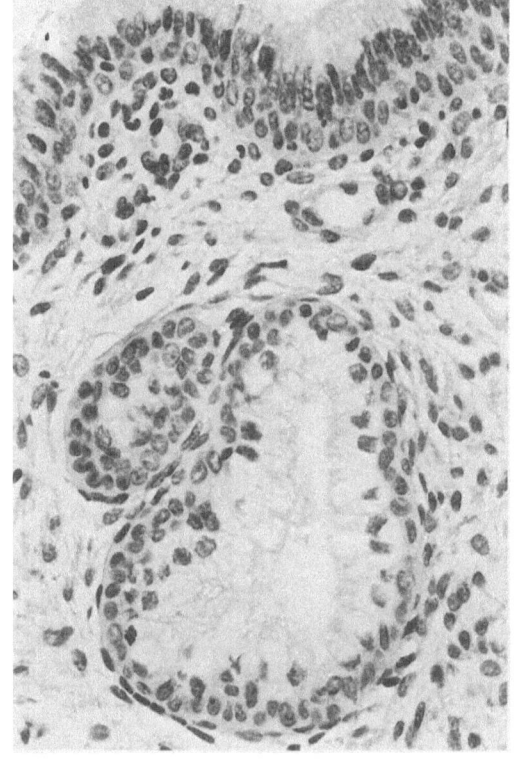

34

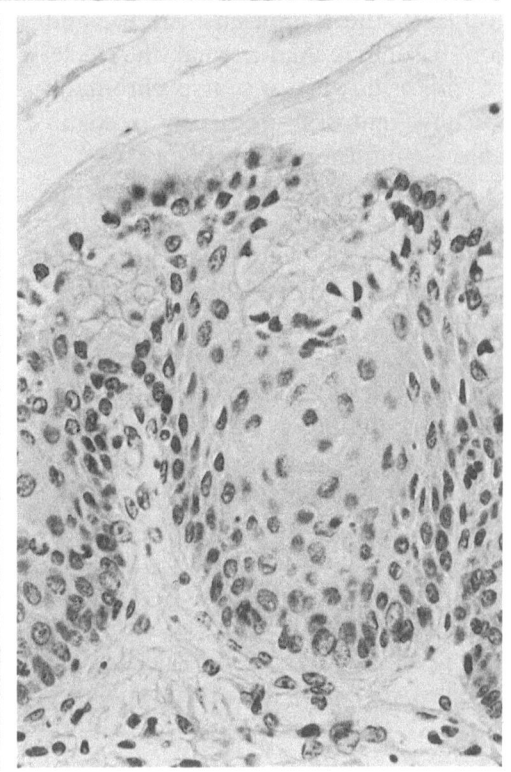

35

Fig. 36. Adenocarcinoma in situ. The endocervical cells display marked atypia. The nuclei are polymorphic, enlarged, and hyperchromatic; some partly atypical mitoses are present. × 335

Fig. 37. Adenocarcinoma in situ. The glandular structures are lined with atypical cells. The cytoplasm is darker and more basophilic than normal, the nuclei are enlarged with a coarse chromatin structure, mitoses are easily recognizable. No infiltrative growth. × 210
This type of lesion is seldom encountered alone. In most cases, it is associated with a CIS, an invasive squamous carcinoma, or an adenocarcinoma.

Fig. 38. Well-differentiated adenocarcinoma of the cervix. About 6%–8% of cervical carcinomas are adenocarcinomas. The neoplastic glandular structures infiltrate the stroma, which is edematous and contains numerous lymphocytes and plasmocytes. Even in poorly differentiated adenocarcinomas, the tumor cells contain some alcian-blue-positive vacuoles (acid mucopolysaccharides). × 335

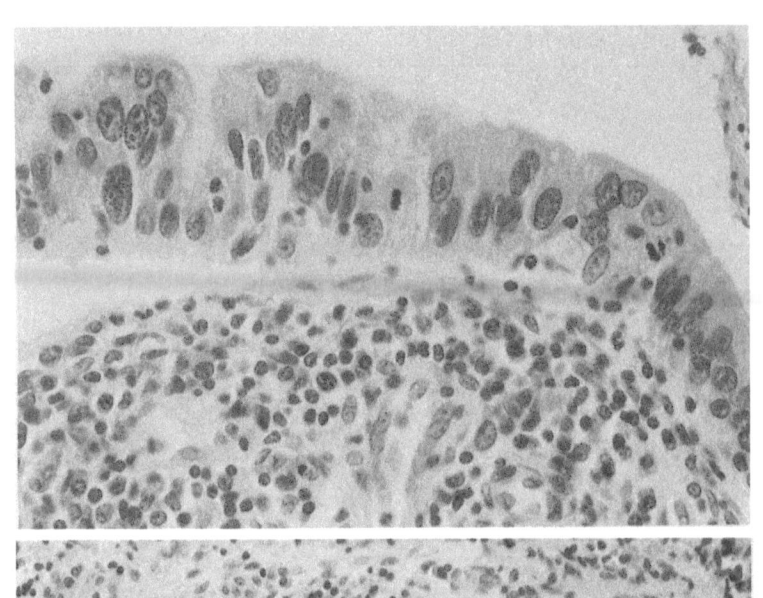

36

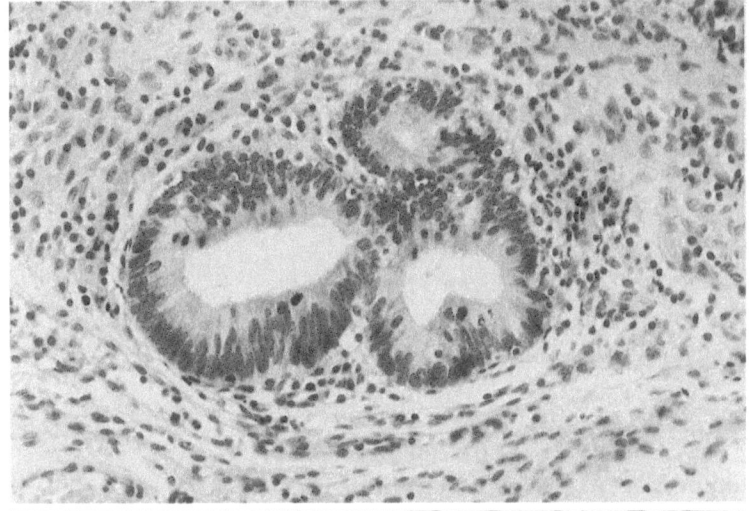

37

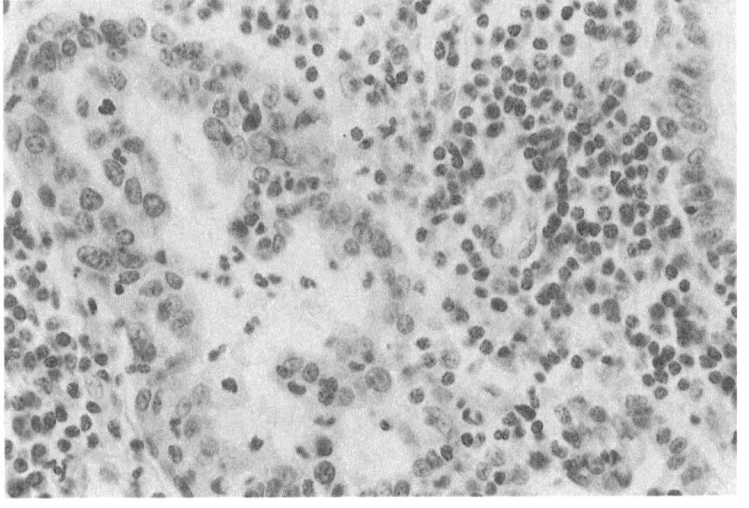

38

Fig. 39. Moderately differentiated cervical squamous cell carcinoma. Large solid strands of tumor cells with individual cell keratinization. The nuclei are markedly polymorphic and contain large nuclei. Partly atypical mitoses are numerous. × 335

Fig. 40. Clear-cell adenocarcinoma. The tumor cells form solid islands and glandular structures. The cell membranes are distinct, the cytoplasm is clear and contains glycogen. The nuclei are polymorphic and hyperchromatic. (× 335) Differential diagnosis: metastatic renal carcinoma!
Such tumors have been repeatedly found in young women after prenatal DES exposure.

Fig. 41. Adenoid cystic carcinoma. Such a tumor is very rare in this location. The microscopic morphology is identical to that of similar tumors in other locations (salivary glands). (× 85) Adenoid cystic carcinoma is locally invasive, distant metastases are uncommon.

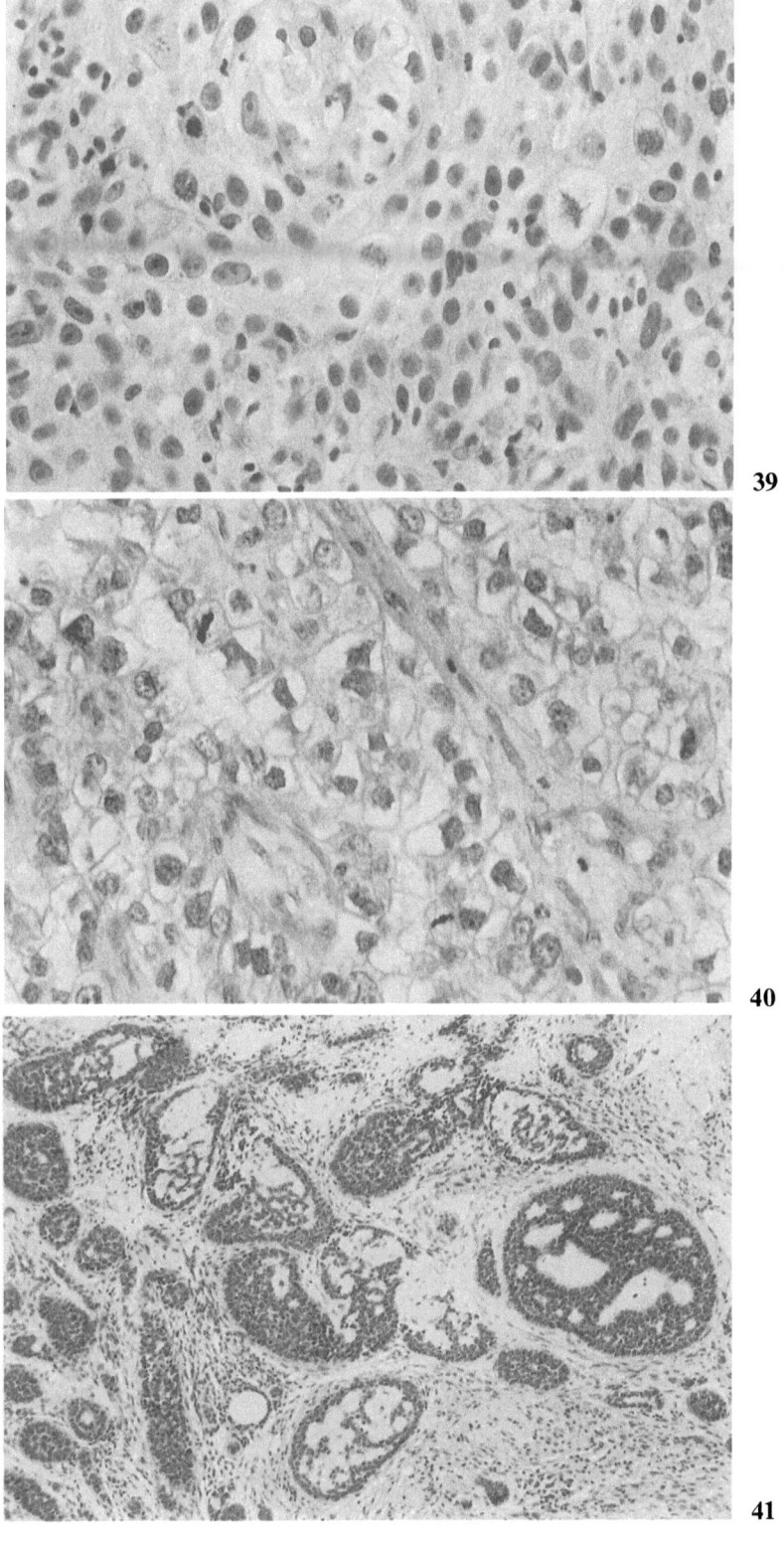

39

40

41

Miscellanous Conditions

Fig. 42. Chronic follicular cervicitis. The surface epithelium is focally exfoliated. The stroma shows edema and lymphocytic and plasmocytic infiltration. A lymphoid follicle is seen near the surface. ×67

Fig. 43. Cervical endometriosis. Endometrial glands in the early secretory phase and endometrial stroma are present under the surface epithelium. ×135

Fig. 44. Decidual transformation of the cervical stroma. The stromal cells may show a marked decidual transformation during pregnancy. They are then enlarged and have distinct cell membranes. The cytoplasm is abundant and eosinophilic. The nuclei are somewhat irregular. ×210

Fig. 45. Microglandular hyperplasia of the cervical glands. This benign condition occurs mostly in women with a history of oral contraceptive use or during and after a pregnancy. It is, therefore, considered to be a result of progestagen stimulation. The glandular units are densely packed together. The epithelial cells are cuboidal with a poor mucus content. The nuclei are somewhat irregular but the nuclear-cytoplasmic ratio is conserved. The poorly developed stroma is infiltrated with leukocytes. ×210
Differential diagnosis: primary adenocarcinoma!

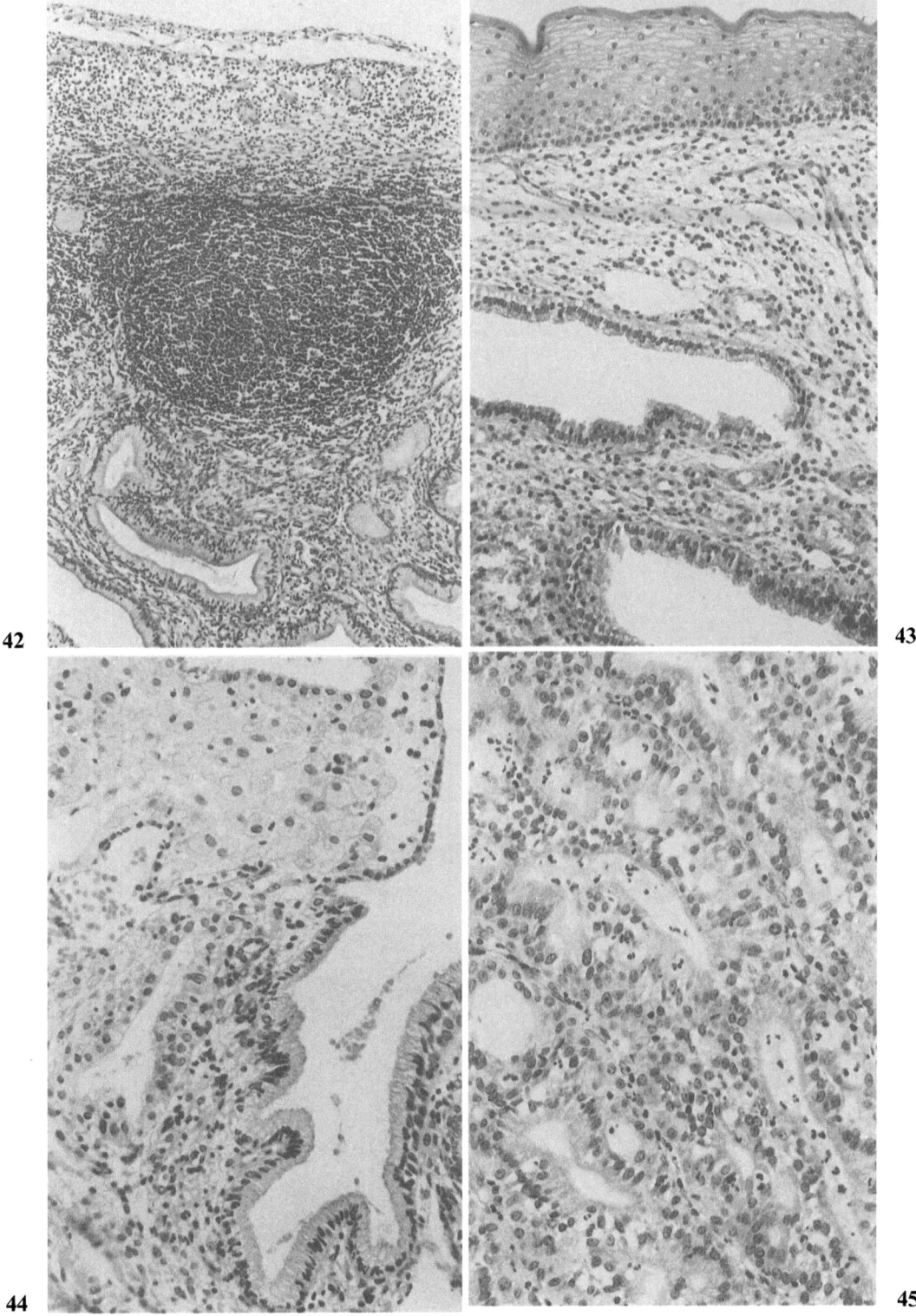

42

43

44

45

IV. Histopathology of the Endometrium

References

Böcker W, Stegner H-E (1975) A light and electron microscopic study of endometrial sarcomas of the uterus. Virchows Arch [Pathol Anat] 368: 141–156

Dallenbach-Hellweg G (1969) Endometrium. Pathologische Histologie in Diagnostik und Forschung. Springer, Berlin Heidelberg New York

Kempson RL, Bari W (1970) Uterine sarcomas. Classification, diagnosis and prognosis. Hum Pathol 1: 331–349

Kurman RJ, Scully RE (1976) Clear cell carcinoma of the endometrium. An analysis of 21 cases. Cancer 37: 872–882

Silverberg SG, Bolin MG, DeGiorgi LS (1972) Adenoacanthoma and mixed adenosquamous carcinoma of the endometrium. Cancer 30: 1307–1314

Fig. 46 A, B. Normal endometrium, early proliferative phase. The endometrium has not thickened yet. The glands are narrow, tubular, and perpendicular to the surface. The glandular epithelium is tall columnar, the nuclei are pseudo-stratified and hyperchromatic. Some mitoses are present. The stroma shows mild edema. *A* ×85; *B* ×336

Fig. 47A, B. Normal endometrium, early secretory phase (3rd day after ovulation). The glands are tortuous, the stroma is edematous. The glandular epithelium is tall columnar and all cells exhibit subnuclear vacuoles, which contain glycogen and displace the nuclei toward the lumen. Mitotic activity may be found until days 3–4 after ovulation. *A* ×85; *B* ×335

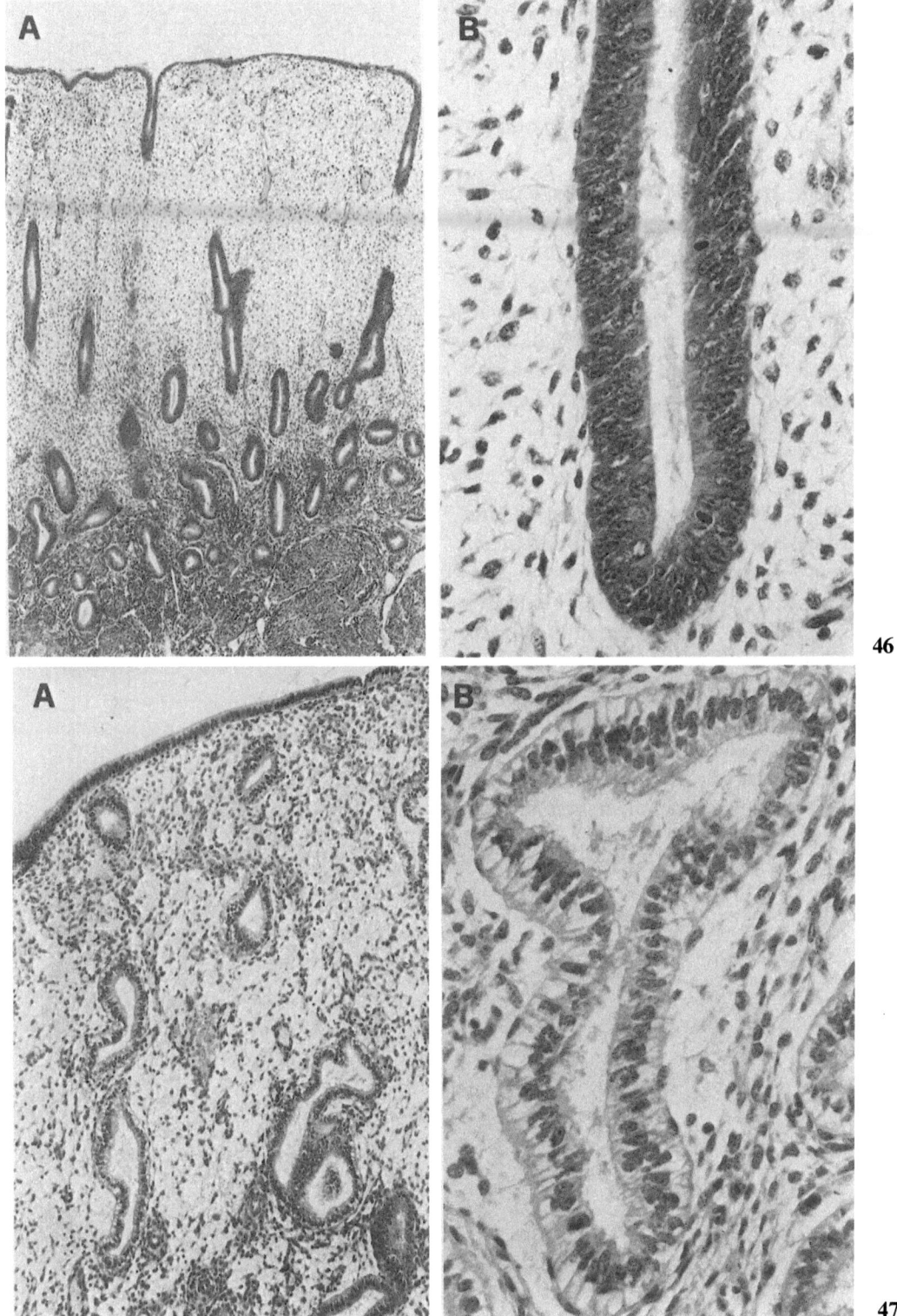

46

47

37

Fig. 48 A, B. Normal endometrium, mid-secretory phase (7 days after ovulation). The stroma is strongly edematous and contains numerous spiral arteries. The glands are tortuous. Because of their secretory activity, the epithelial cells have indistinct and frayed luminal borders. The nuclei are basally located. *A* ×85; *B* ×335

Fig. 49 A, B. Normal endometrium, late secretory phase (11 days after ovulation). The predecidual transformation of the stromal cells, which begins around the spiral arteries and under the surface epithelium, now affects all stromal cells. Spiral arteries are noted under the surface epithelium accompanied by dilated and thin-walled blood vessels. The glands began to collapse, the secretory activity of the glandular cells is greatly decreased. *A* ×85; *B* ×335

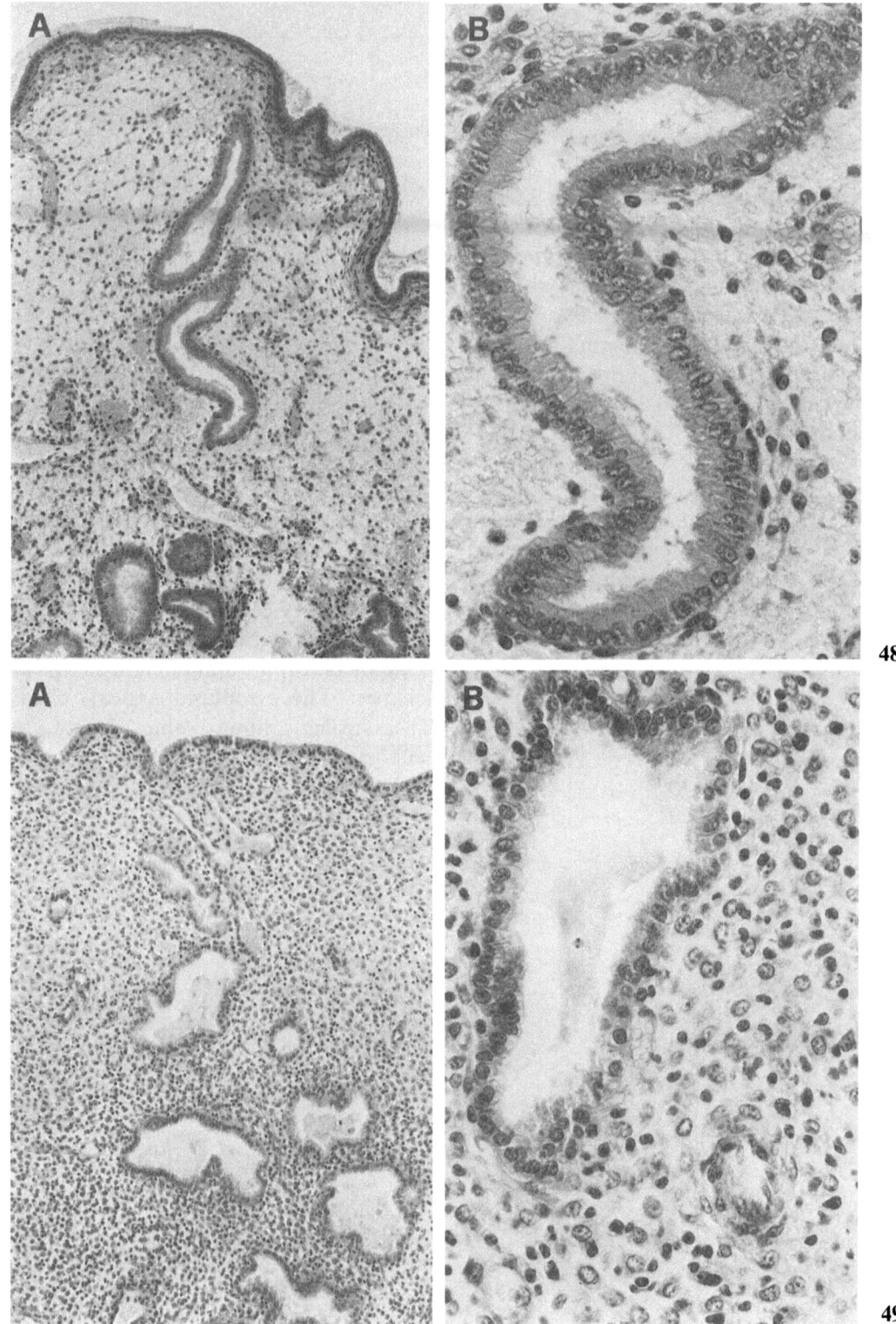

48

49

Fig. 50 A, B. Endometrium after several cycles of oral contraceptives (in this case, Anacyclin 101, a progestin-dominated preparation). The stroma shows a considerable pseudodecidual transformation and a discrete lymphocytic infiltration. Glands are few in number, small, and lined with low inactive epithelium. *A* ×85; *B* ×335

Fig. 51. Endometrium during inadequate luteal phase. This curettage was performed on postovulation day 8. The stroma shows only mild edema. Some epithelial cells exhibit subnuclear vacuoles and the glandular lumina show very little secretion. ×335

Fig. 52. Endometrium after spontaneous abortion (so-called Arias-Stella phenomenon). The endometrial glands are hypersecretory and the epithelium forms small papillae. The nuclei are quite pleomorphic and often in an apical location. The cytoplasm appears clear. The stroma shows some degree of leukocytic infiltration. ×110
Differential diagnosis: clear-cell adenocarcinoma!

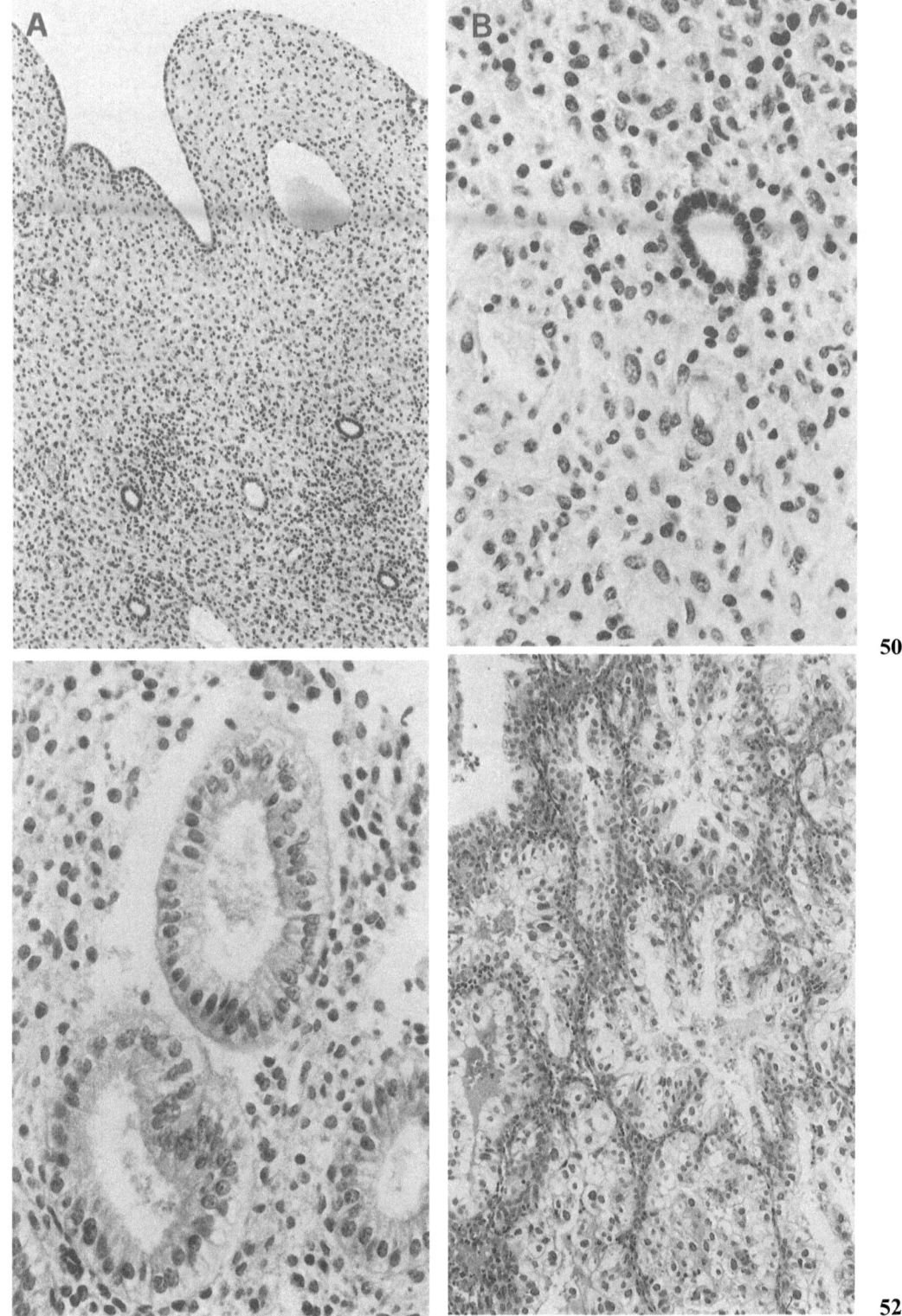

Fig. 53. Nonspecific endometritis. The stroma is edematous and shows a severe leukocytic infiltration. The glandular epithelium may occasionally be hyperplastic but displays no functional activity. Leukocytes may disrupt the glands and fill their lumina. ×250
The diagnosis of chronic nonspecific endometritis relies on the identification of plasmocytes. Lymphocytes and lymphoid follicles also occur in normal endometrium.

Fig. 54A, B. Tuberculous endometritis. The glandular epithelium may be hyperplastic but never displays any functional activity. Numerous granulomas with Langhans' giant cells are found in the stroma, which also shows lymphocytic infiltration. A central caseous necrosis of the granulomas is rarely present. As in nonspecific endometritis, the inflammation may destroy the endometrial glands. A diagnostic curettage for tuberculous endometritis must be performed shortly before menstruation. As the lesion is often only focally developed, the whole uterine cavity must be curetted. *A* ×85; *B* ×210

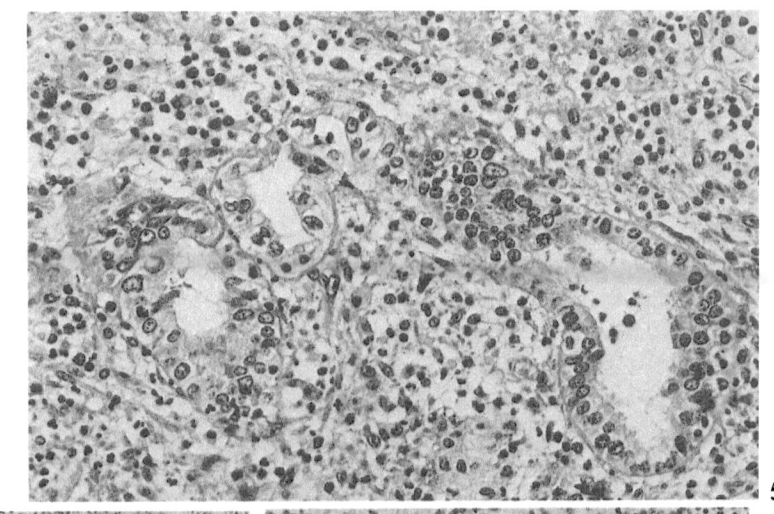

53

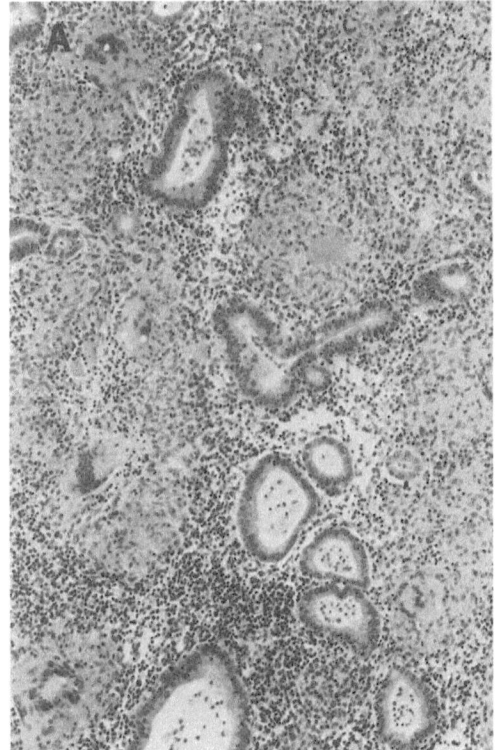

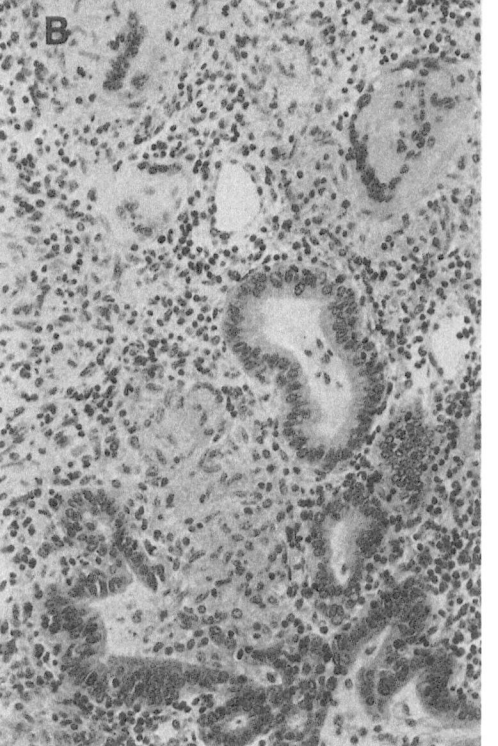

54

Fig. 55 A, B. Glandular-cystic hyperplasia. The endometrium is thickened and often polypoid. The stroma is occasionally edematous and contains dilated blood vessels. The glands are numerous. They may be tightly packed and/or cystic (Swiss cheese pattern). The glandular epithelium is tall columnar with enlarged hyperchromatic nuclei. Mitosic activity is often present to a moderate extent. *A* ×85; *B* ×335

Such a condition represents a response to exogenous or endogenous estrogenic hyperstimulation.

Fig. 56. Atypical adenomatous hyperplasia. The glands are numerous and highly hyperplastic with very little intervening stroma. The glandular epithelium is often strongly eosinophilic and forms small intraluminal papillae. The nuclei are enlarged, pleomorphic, and exhibit prominent nucleoli. Mitoses are numerous. ×210

The lack of a "dos-à-dos" pattern and absence of infiltration permit this lesion to be distinguished from well-differentiated adenocarcinoma.

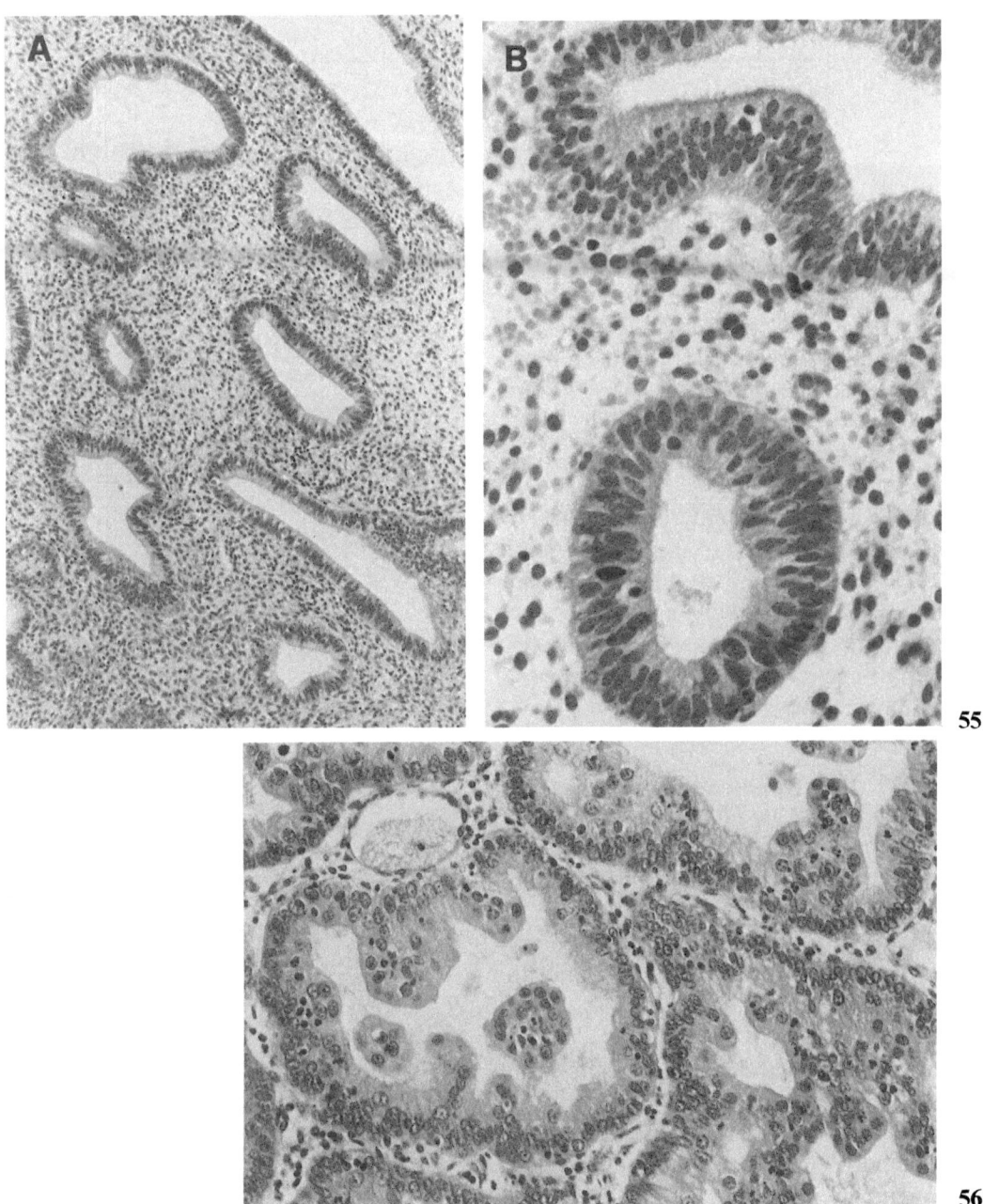

55

56

Fig. 57. Well-differentiated endometrial adenocarcinoma (grade 1). The glands are tightly packed and exhibit numerous "dos-à-dos" patterns. The glandular epithelium consists of one or more cell layers. The nuclei are enlarged and moderately pleomorphic. ×210

Fig. 58. Moderately differentiated adenocarcinoma (grade 2). The tumor tissue consists of glandular structures and solid areas. ×210. The well- and moderately differentiated endometrial adenocarcinoma have a marked tendency toward exophytic growth.

Fig. 59. Poorly differentiated adenocarcinoma (grade 3). The tumor tissue consists almost exclusively of solid epithelial proliferations. Glandular structures are rarely seen. ×210
The poorly differentiated adenocarcinoma tends to invade rapidly into the myometrium.
The grade of differentiation of endometrial adenocarcinomas may be quite different from one area to another. It is, therefore, important to examine many specimens of tumor tissue. Some anaplastic carcinomas may be difficult to distinguish from high-grade endometrial stromal sarcoma. In such cases, a reticulin stain may help to achieve a differential diagnosis. The depth of invasion in the myometrium is an important prognostic factor together with the grade of differentiation. All pathology reports should mention both!

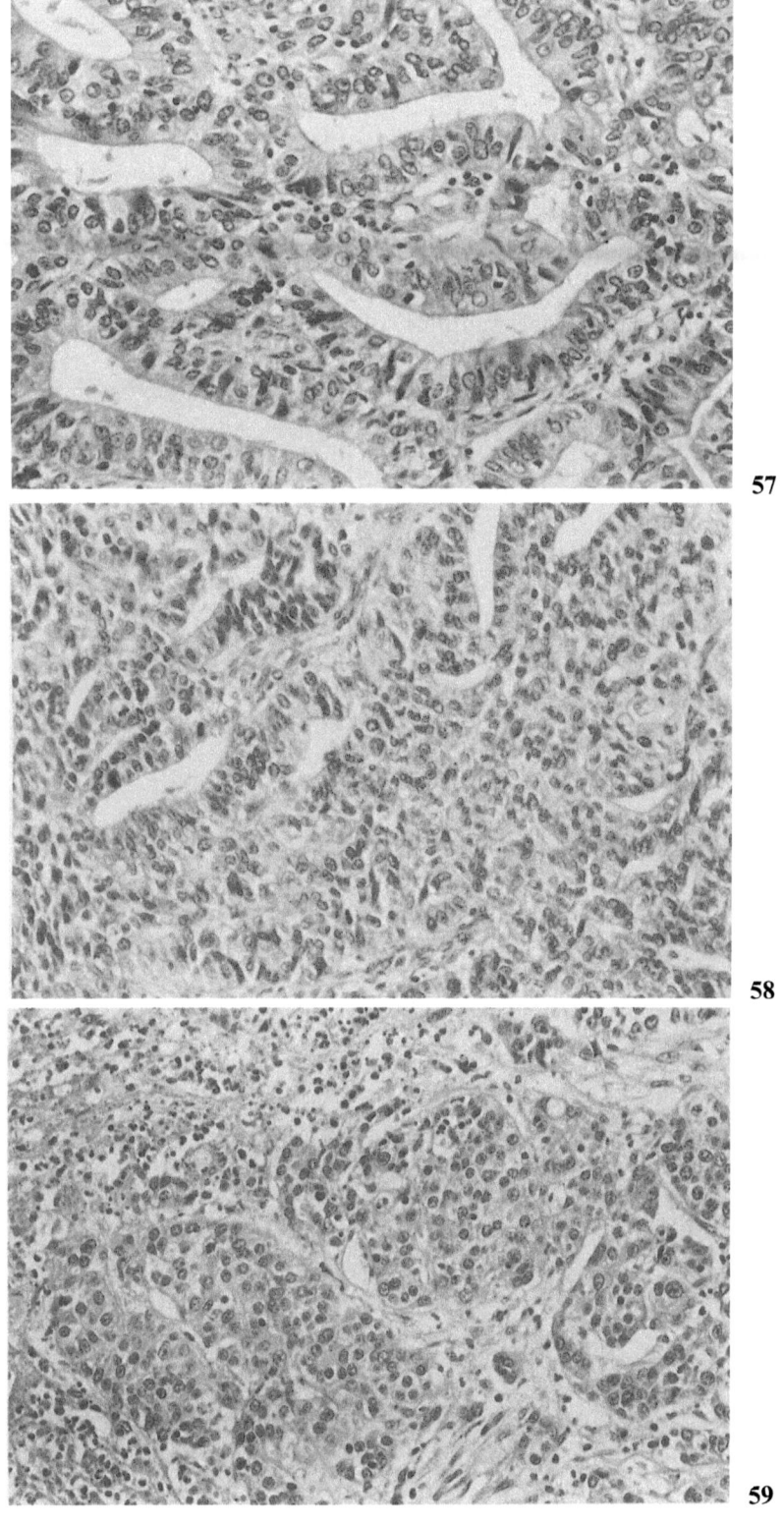

57

58

59

Fig. 60. Adenocarcinoma with squamous differentiation. They are mostly well-differentiated adenocarcinomas, which contain substantial amounts of squamous epithelium, often with keratin formation. ×210

The prognosis of such tumors is identical to that of adenocarcinomas of the same grade without squamous differentiation.

Fig. 61. Papillary and focal clear-cell adenocarcinoma. This is a particular type of well-differentiated endometrial carcinoma, which tends to show exophytic growth. ×135

Fig. 62. Clear-cell adenocarcinoma. This type of carcinoma is characterized by cells with clear cytoplasm arranged in solid masses with papillary and tubular patterns. The cell membranes are distinct, the nuclei are pleomorphic. ×210

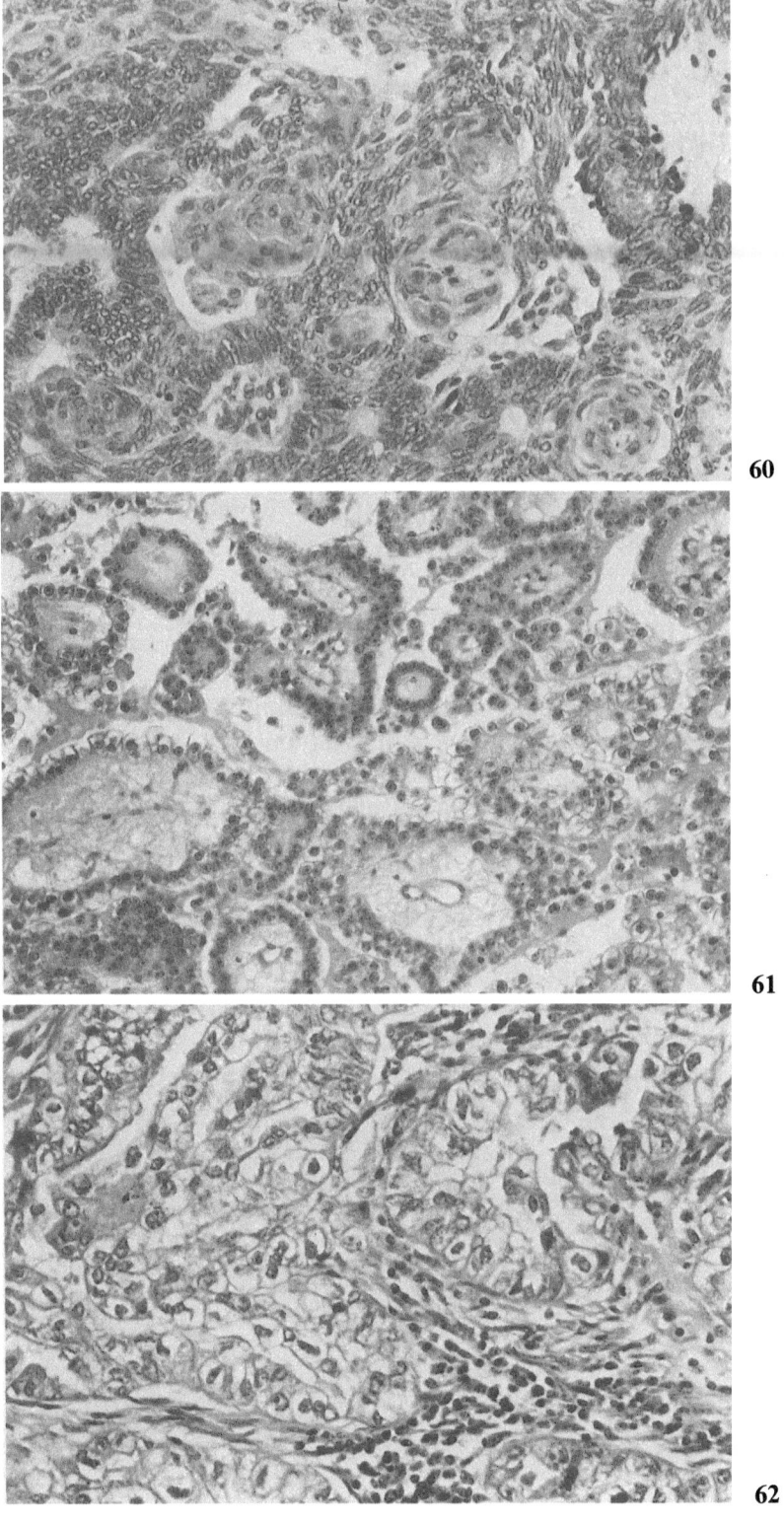

60

61

62

Malignant Mixed Mesodermal Tumors

This tumor type is relatively rare and occurs mostly in elderly women. A disproportionate number of such tumors develop after pelvic irradiation. Similar extrauterine tumors are believed to arise in foci of endometriosis. Histologically, these tumors consist of carcinomatous glands within a sarcomatous stroma, both elements being sharply separated by a basement membrane (Fig. 63).

In the homologous tumors, also called carcinosarcomas, the sarcomatous element represents fibrosarcoma, endometrial stromal sarcoma, or leiomyosarcoma. In the heterologous tumors, the sarcomatous components are most frequently rhabdomyoblasts and cartilage. Less common heterologous elements are osteoid, bone, and fat (Figs. 64, 65).

Fig. 63 A–C. Homologous malignant mixed mesodermal tumor (so-called carcinosarcoma). The carcinomatous glands and the sarcomatous stroma are both easily recognizable and distinguishable from one another. *A* ×210; *B* ×270; *C* reticulin stain ×270

Fig. 64. Heterologous malignant mixed mesodermal tumor. In this case, numerous areas consisting of neoplastic cartilage are present. ×135

Fig. 65. Heterologous malignant mixed mesodermal tumor. Numerous well-differentiated rhabdomyoblasts with distinct cross-striations are present in the sarcomatous stroma. ×335

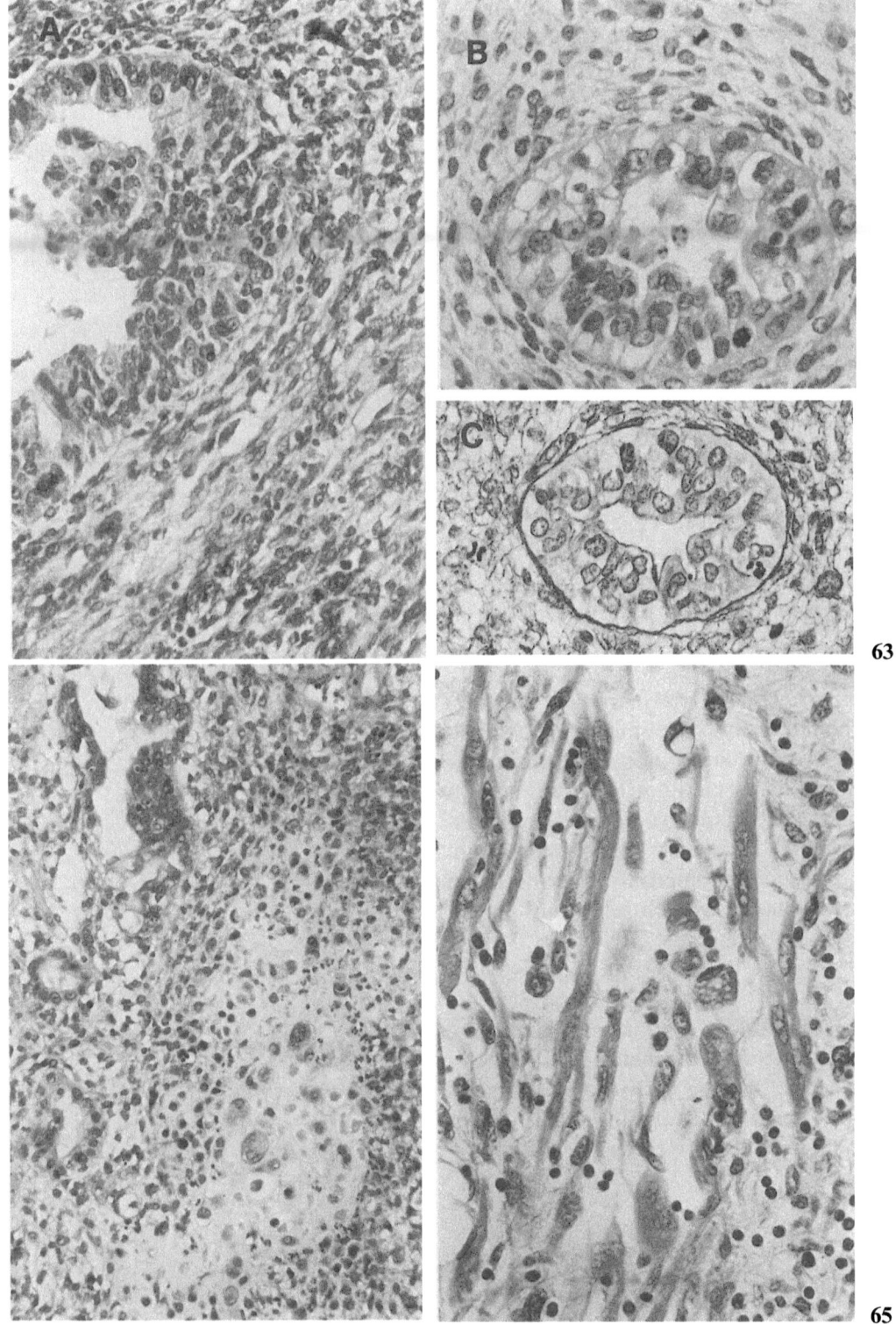

63

64

65

Fig. 66. Stromatosis (stromal endo-metriosis, endolymphatic stromatosis, low-grade endometrial stromal sar-coma). This lesion is characterized by masses of cells resembling stromal cells of the proliferating endometrium, which invade the myometrium. Invasion of lymphatic and vascular channels is typi-cal for this lesion. The tumor cells show little variation in size and shape, the nuclei are round to oval, the nucleoli are inconspicuous. × 135

The exact histogenesis and nature of this rare condition as well as its treat-ment are still under discussion.

Fig. 67. Endometrial stromal sarcoma. The tumors cells are spindle-shaped and display pleomorphic hyperchromatic nuclei. Partly pathologic mitoses are nu-merous. Reticulin stain may be neces-sary to distinguish this lesion from anaplastic endometrial carcinoma. In stromal sarcoma, each cell is surrounded by reticulin fibers. × 210

Fig. 68. Serous ovarian carcinoma me-tastatic to the endometrium. The endo-metrium is in the early secretory phase. The lymphatics contain small groups of tumor cells as well as a few lympho-cytes. × 210

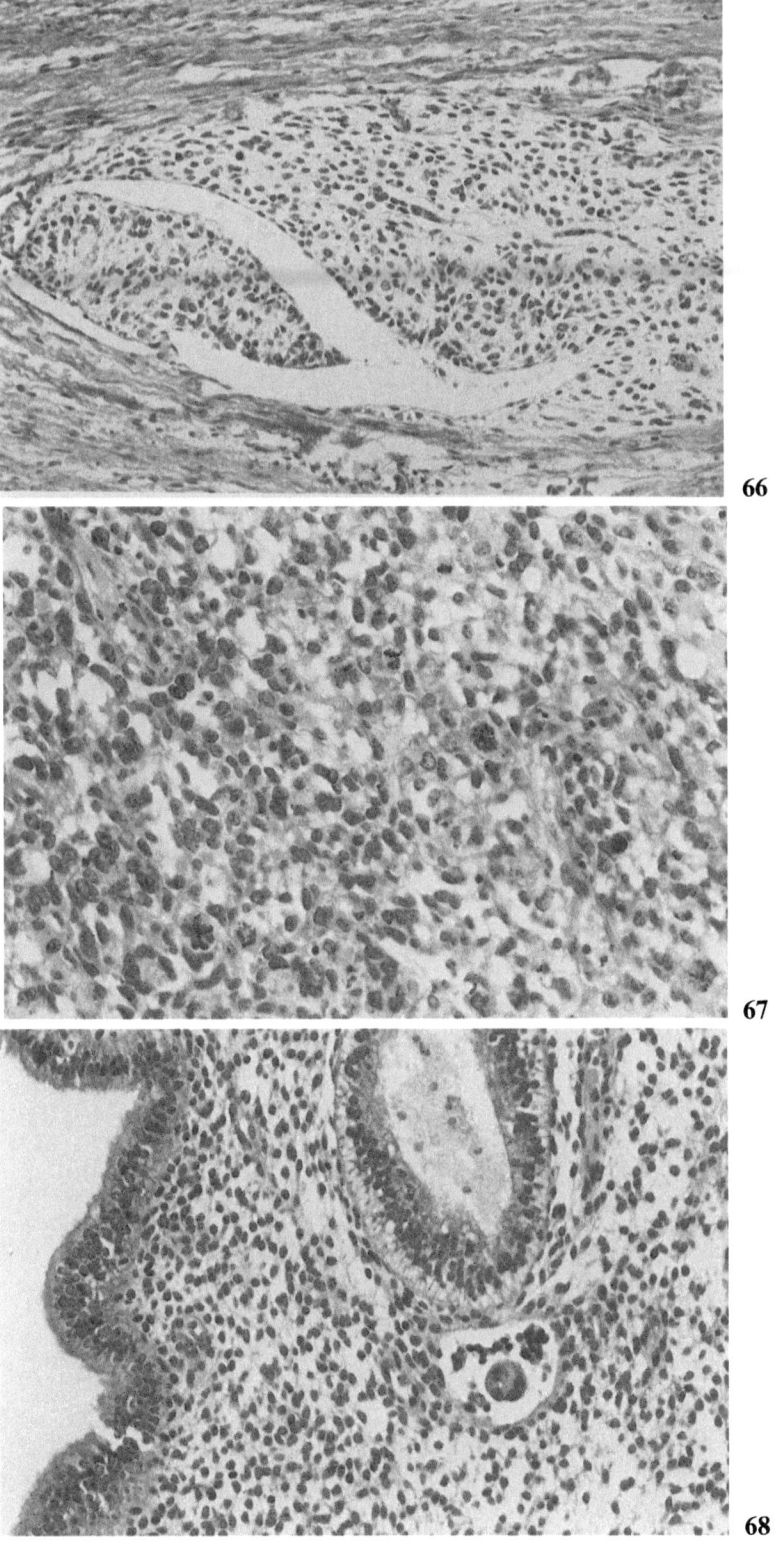

66

67

68

V. Histopathology of the Myometrium

References

Abell MR, Littler ER (1975) Benign metastasizing uterine leiomyoma. Cancer 36: 2206–2213

Gupta RK, Hunter RE (1964) Lipoma of the uterus: review of literature with views on histogenesis. Obstet Gynecol 24:255–257

Jacobs DS, Cohen H, Johnson JS (1965) Lipoleiomyomas of the uterus. Am J Clin Pathol 44:45–51

Kempson RL, Bari W (1970) Uterine sarcomas. Classification, diagnosis, and prognosis. Hum Pathol 1:331–349

Saksela E, Lampinen V, Procopé B-J (1974) Malignant mesenchymal tumors of the uterine corpus. Am J Obstet Gynecol 120: 452–460

Taylor HB, Norris HJ (1966) Mesenchymal tumors of the uterus. IV. Diagnosis and prognosis of leiomyosarcoma. Arch Pathol Lab Med 82:40–44

Williams LJ, Pavlick FJ (1980) Leiomyomatosis peritonealis disseminata: two case reports and a review of the medical literature. Cancer 45:1726–1733

Fig. 69. Adenomyosis (endometriosis interna). Numerous endometrial glands surrounded by endometrial stroma are present in the myometrium. Usually, the endometrial epithelium shows no cyclic changes. ×42

Fig. 70. "Myometritis syncytialis". During normal pregnancy, some trophoblastic giant cells may invade the myometrium and uterine veins. Only a single giant-cell invasion is seen in this condition, in contrast to choriocarcinoma in which large masses of cyto- and syncytiotrophoblastic cells invade and destroy the myometrium with accompanying necrosis and hemorrhage. ×135

Fig. 71. Hemangioma. This is a rare benign tumor in the myometrium. It is not encapsulated and poorly demarcated. Numerous thin-walled vessels filled with erythrocytes are tightly packed. ×53

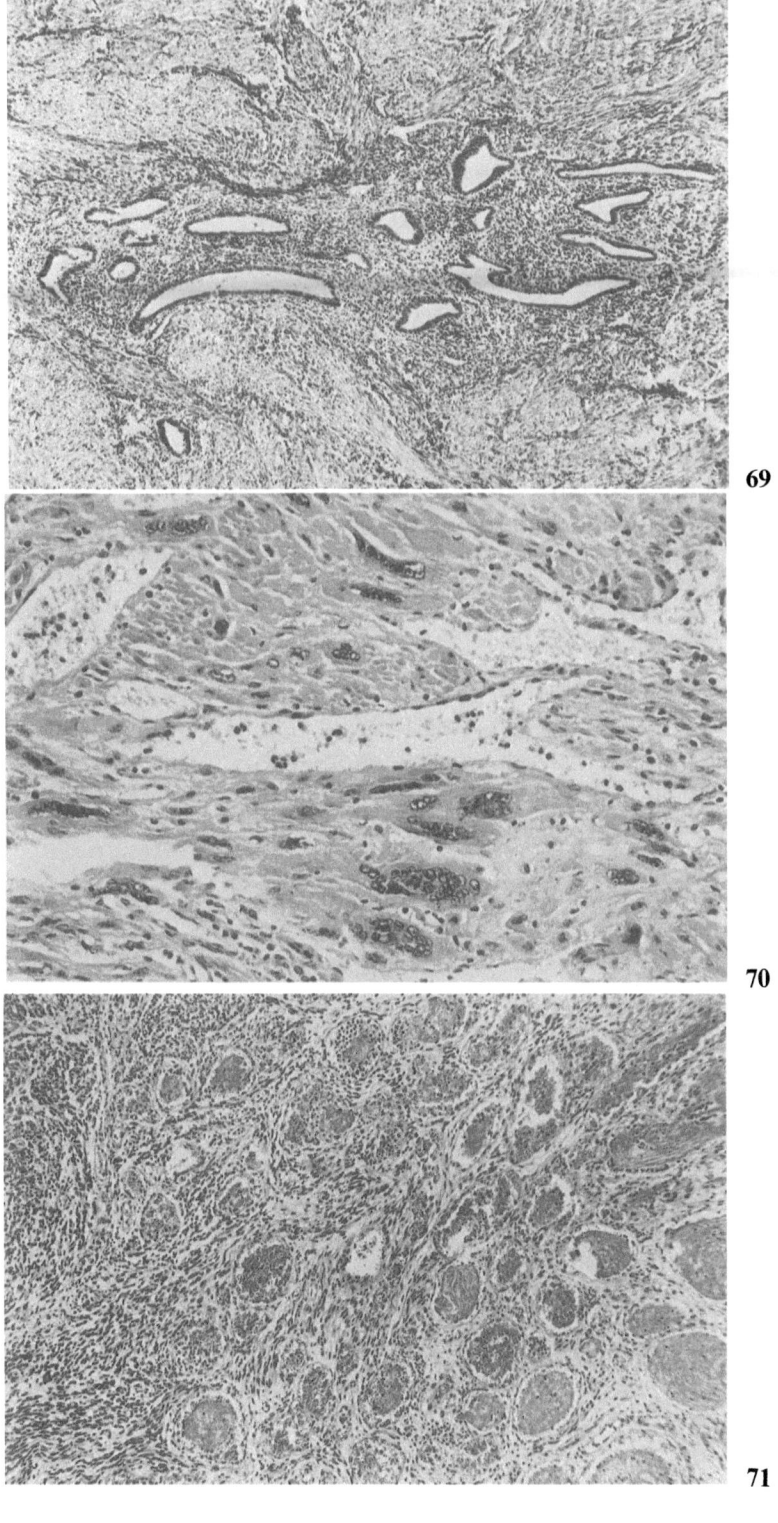

69

70

71

Fig. 72. Lipoma of the uterus. Pure lipomas are very rare in this location. Their gross and microscopic characteristics are the same as those of lipomas in other locations. × 85

Fig. 73. Lipoleiomyoma of the uterus. This tumor type is more common than the pure lipoma. Microscopically, it is composed of fat tissue mixed with bundles of smooth muscle cells. × 85

Fig. 74. Leiomyoma. This benign tumor is very common in the uterine wall. The question whether these neoplasms develop from the smooth muscle cells of the myometrium or blood vessels is still under discussion. Estrogens may stimulate their growth. During pregnancy, leiomyomas develop often considerable regressive changes, which can lead to total necrosis of the tumor. Microscopically, the leiomyomas are composed of interlacing bundles of smooth muscle cells admixed with more or less connective tissue and collagen fibers (fibroleiomyoma). × 135

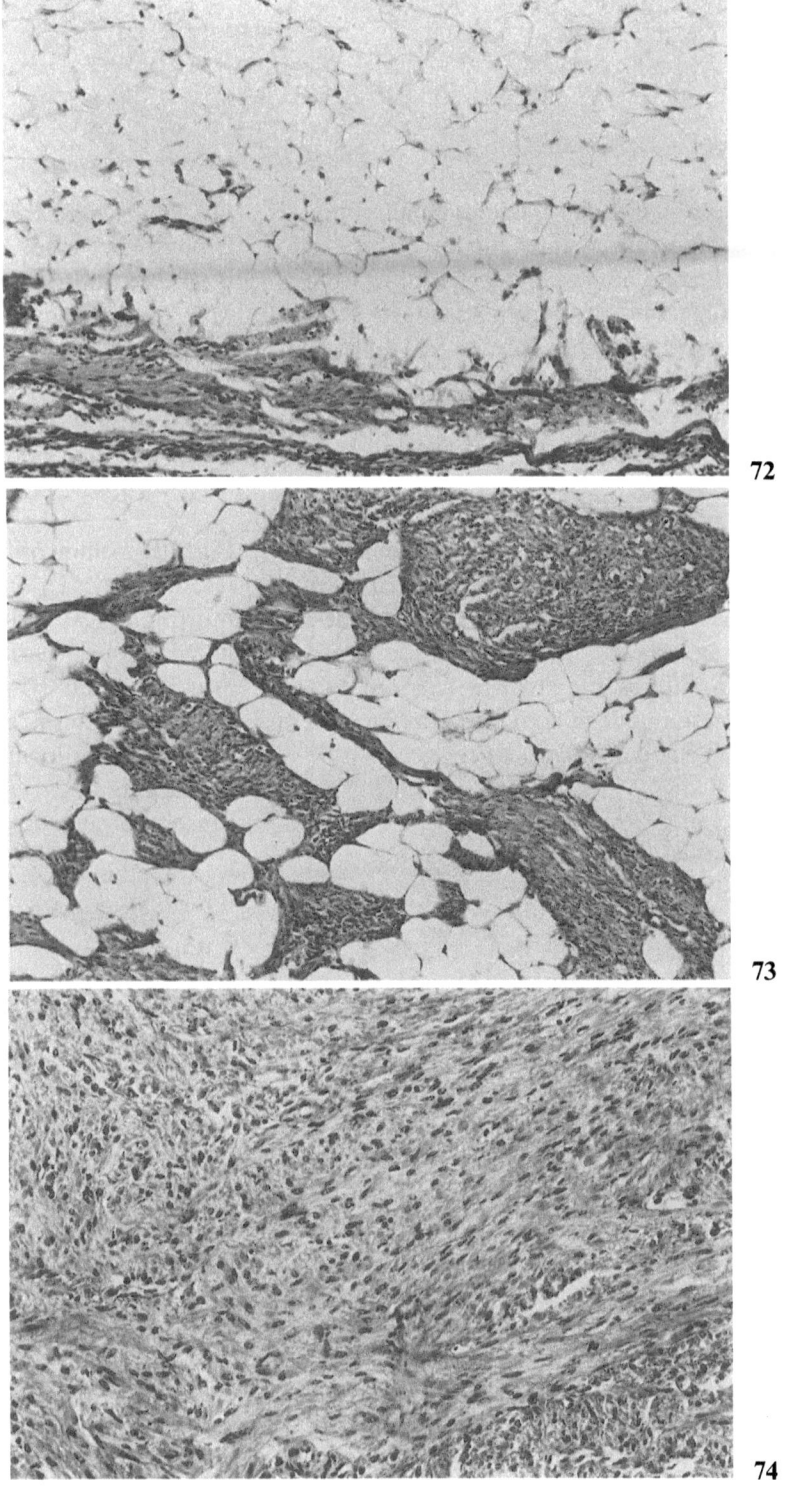

72

73

74

Fig. 75. Cellular leiomyoma. In this benign tumor, the cells have scant cytoplasm. The nuclei are round to oval with a fine chromatin structure. Normal mitoses may be present in small number. ×210
Differential diagnosis: low-grade leiomyosarcoma!

Fig. 76. Symplastic leiomyoma. Some leiomyomas may present focally considerable cellular and nuclear changes. Many cells are multinucleated, the nuclei are often hyperchromatic but no mitoses are present. ×135

Fig. 77. Symplastic leiomyoma. The development of the symplastic giant cells is probably due to regressive changes. The nuclear and cellular abnormalities may cause concern but as long as mitotic activity is low or absent, they have no significance. ×210

Fig. 78. Leiomyoblastoma (epitheloid leiomyoma). This tumor is rare and no morphological criteria permit its behavior to be predicted. The tumor cells are polygonal with distinct cell membranes. The nuclei are round to oval and centrally located. The cytoplasm is abundant and vacuolated and often presents a perinuclear halo. ×335

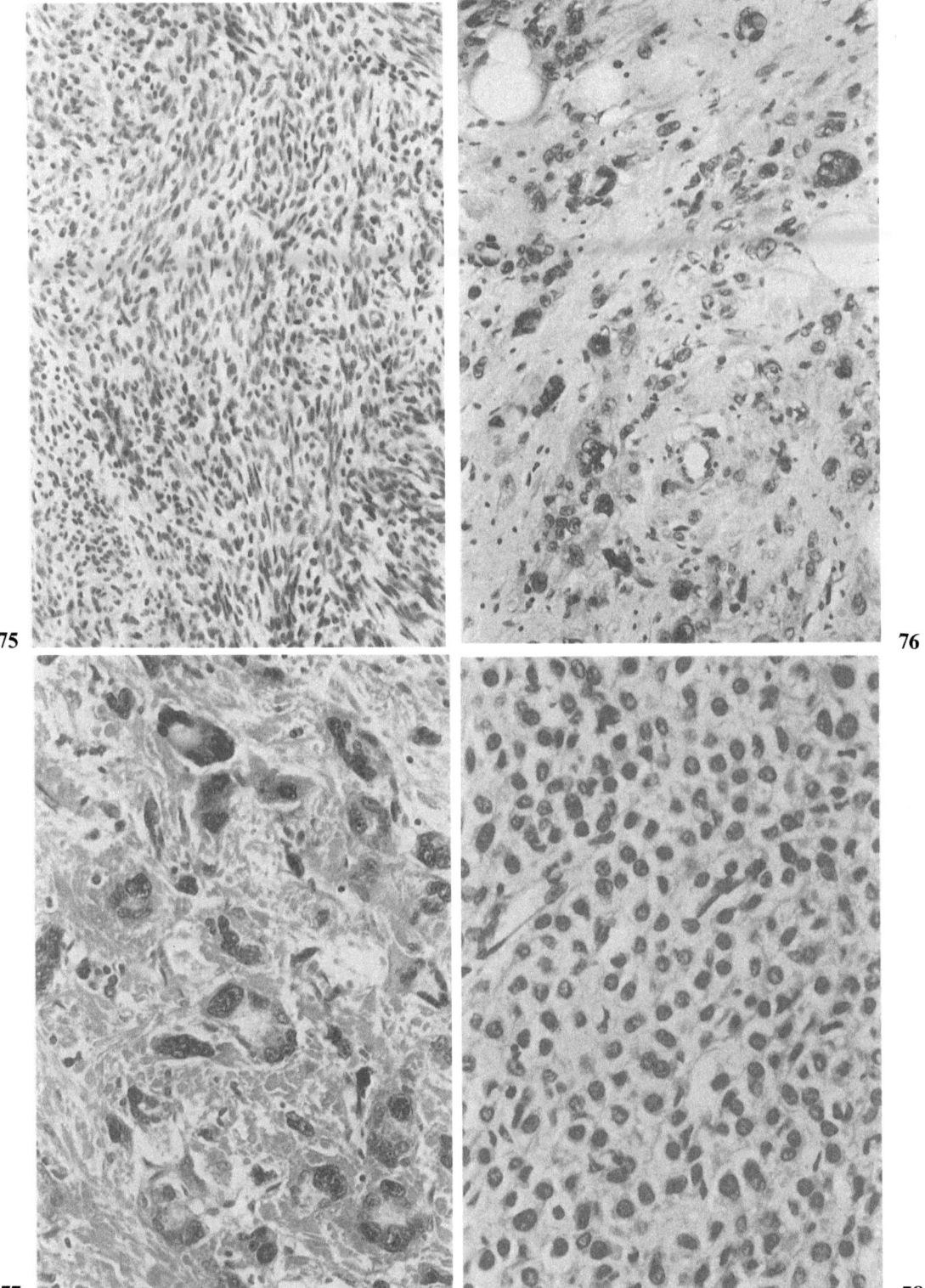

75

76

77

78

61

Fig. 79. Leiomyosarcoma. This malignant tumor of the myometrium is uncommon (about 1 leiomyosarcoma/50 endometrial carcinomas) and develops hematogenous metastases. Microscopically, the tumor is composed of bundles of spindle-shaped cells with elongated, pleomorphic, and hyperchromatic nuclei. The presence of ten or more mitotic figures/ten high-power fields (HPF) is diagnostic of leiomyosarcoma. ×210

Fig. 80. Leiomyosarcoma. In this tumor, there is palisading of the nuclei quite reminiscent of the pattern seen in neurinomas. ×53

Fig. 81. Gastric carcinoma metastatic to the myometrium. The lymphatic vessels in the myometrium contain numerous carcinomatous cells, which occasionally form small glandular structures. ×335

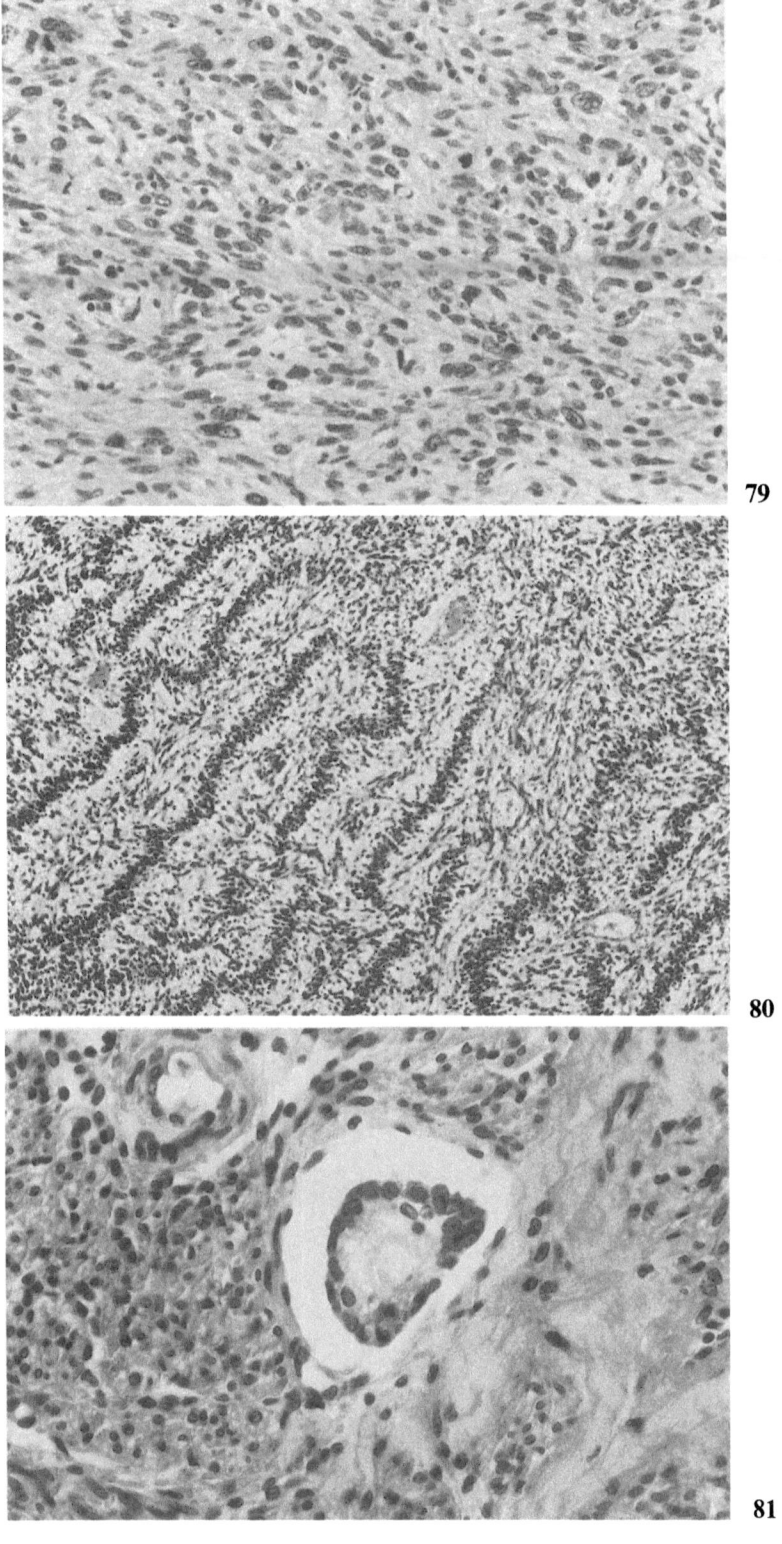

79

80

81

63

VI. Histopathology of the Fallopian Tube

References

Novak ER, Woodruff JD (1974) Novak's gynecologic and obstetric pathology, 7th edn. Saunders, Philadelphia, pp 288–327

Salazar H, Kanbour A, Burgess F (1972) Ultrastructure and observations on the histogenesis of mesotheliomas "adenomatoid tumors" of the female genital tract. Cancer 29: 141–152

Fig. 82. Acute nonspecific salpingitis. The mucosal folds are strongly edematous and show severe leukocytic infiltration. The surface epithelium may be destroyed but can also occasionally exhibit some degree of hyperplasia. The lumen is filled with an inflammatory exsudate and cellular detritus. × 335

Fig. 83. Chronic nonspecific salpingitis. The plicae of the mucosa adhere to one another. Their stroma shows some degree of fibrosis and chronic inflammation. The surface epithelium is intact, sometimes hyperplastic. × 53

Fig. 84. Tuberculous salpingitis. The folds of the mucosa are broad and adhere to one another. Their stroma contains numerous granulomas with and without central caseous necrosis, some Langhans' giant cells, and lymphocytic infiltrates. × 85

Fig. 85. Foreign-body reaction after hysterosalpingography. The histologic features resemble those of tuberculous salpingitis but there is no necrosis, the giant cells are of a foreign-body type, they lie mostly in the center of the granulomas and often contain visible foreign bodies (▷). × 135

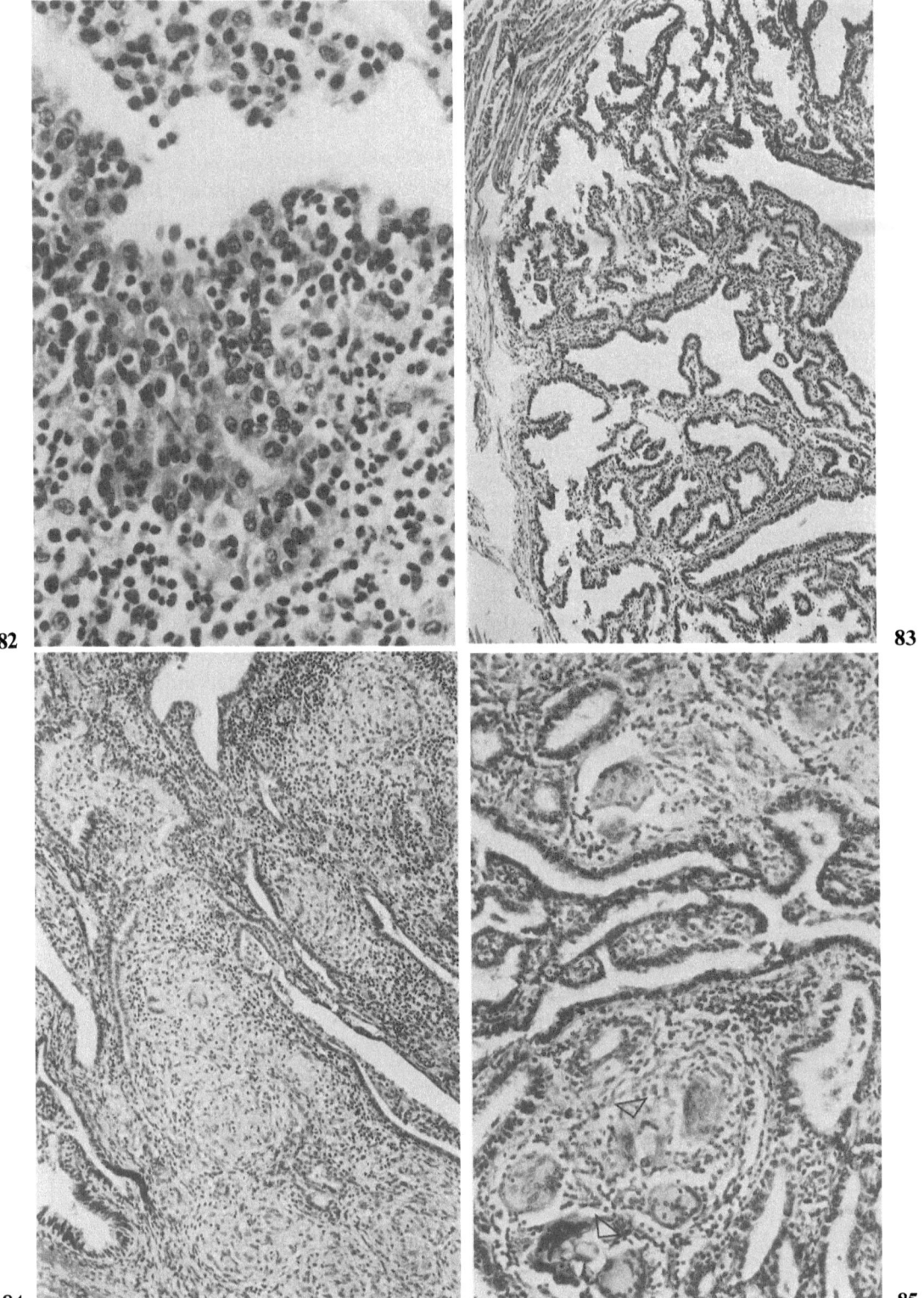

82

83

84

85

Fig. 86. Ruptured tubal pregnancy. The muscle wall of the tube is edematous and infiltrated by leukocytes. The mucosa has been destroyed by the placental villi, which can be seen in the lumen. Practically no decidua is present. × 42

Fig. 87. Decidual transformation of the tubal mucosa. During normal pregnancy, the stromal cells in the tubal mucosa may show decidual transformation. The decidual cells are large with distinct cell borders and abundant eosinophilic cytoplasm. × 170

Fig. 88. Carcinoma of the fallopian tube. The normal mucosa is replaced by a predominantly solid and invasive growing tumor tissue. × 85
Tubal carcinoma is a rare malignancy. Its histologic features are very similar to those of ovarian carcinoma. When the tumor involves both the fallopian tube and ovary, it may be impossible to decide whether the carcinoma is a tubal or ovarian primary malignancy.

Fig. 89. Adenomatoid tumor of the fallopian tube (benign mesothelioma). This benign tumor is grossly and microscopically sharply demarcated and appears as a small nodule under the tubal serosa. Histologically, it is composed of multiple tubular or slitlike structures lined with cuboidal or flattened epithelium with scant intervening stroma. × 210

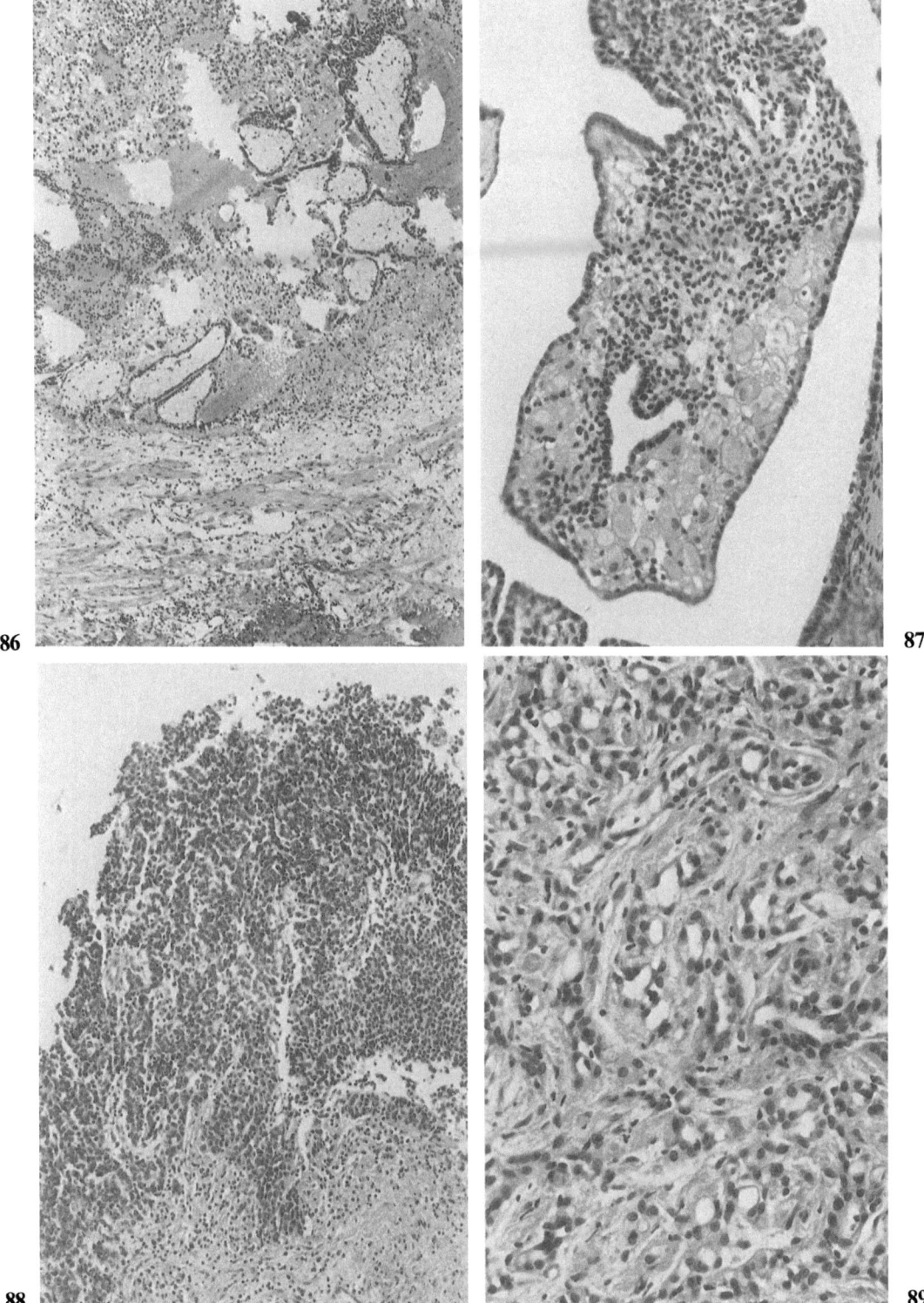

86

87

88

89

VII. Histopathology of the Ovary

References

International Federation of Gynecology and Obstetrics (1971) Classification and staging of malignant tumours in the female pelvis. Acta Obstet Gynecol Scand 50: 1–7

Marchewsky AM, Kaneko M (1978) Bilateral ovarian endometriosis associated with carcinosarcoma of the right ovary and endometrioid carcinoma of the left ovary. Am J Clin Pathol 70: 709–712

Morris JMcL, Scully RE (1958) Endocrine pathology of the ovary. Mosby, St. Louis

Scully RE (1979) Tumors of the ovary and maldeveloped gonads. Atlas of tumor pathology, 2nd series, Fascicle 16. Armed Forces Institute of Pathology, Washington DC

Serov SF, Scully RE (1973) Histological typing of ovarian tumors. International histological classification of tumours No. 9. Geneva, World Health Organization

Teilum G (1971) Special tumors of ovary and testis and related extragonadal lesions. Comparative pathology and histological identification. Munksgaard, Copenhagen

Fig. 90. Polycystic ovary. The cortex of the ovary is thickened by fibrous tissue and contains numerous primitive follicles. The graafian follicles are cystic and both granulosal and thecal cell layers are hyperplastic. The theca cells may be luteinized. × 53

This condition is most commonly associated with an intermittent or persistent anovulatory syndrome. It may lead to virilism.

Fig. 91. Cystic follicle and involutional corpus luteum. The cystic follicle (*lower half*) is lined with a few layers of granulosa and theca cells. The cystic involutional corpus luteum (*upper half*) contains fibrin, which covers the granulation tissue and luteinized theca cells. × 85

Fig. 92. Hilus (Leydig's) cells. The hilus cells are large with abundant cytoplasm, which may contain crystals of Reinke and/or lipochrome pigments. The nuclei are round with a prominent eccentric nucleolus. These cells are commonly in close apposition to nerve fibers and small blood vessels in the ovarian hilus. × 335

Fig. 93. Hyperthecosis. The ovarian stroma is focally or diffusely hyperplastic and displays multiple foci of luteinized stromal cells. × 210

This condition may cause virilism.

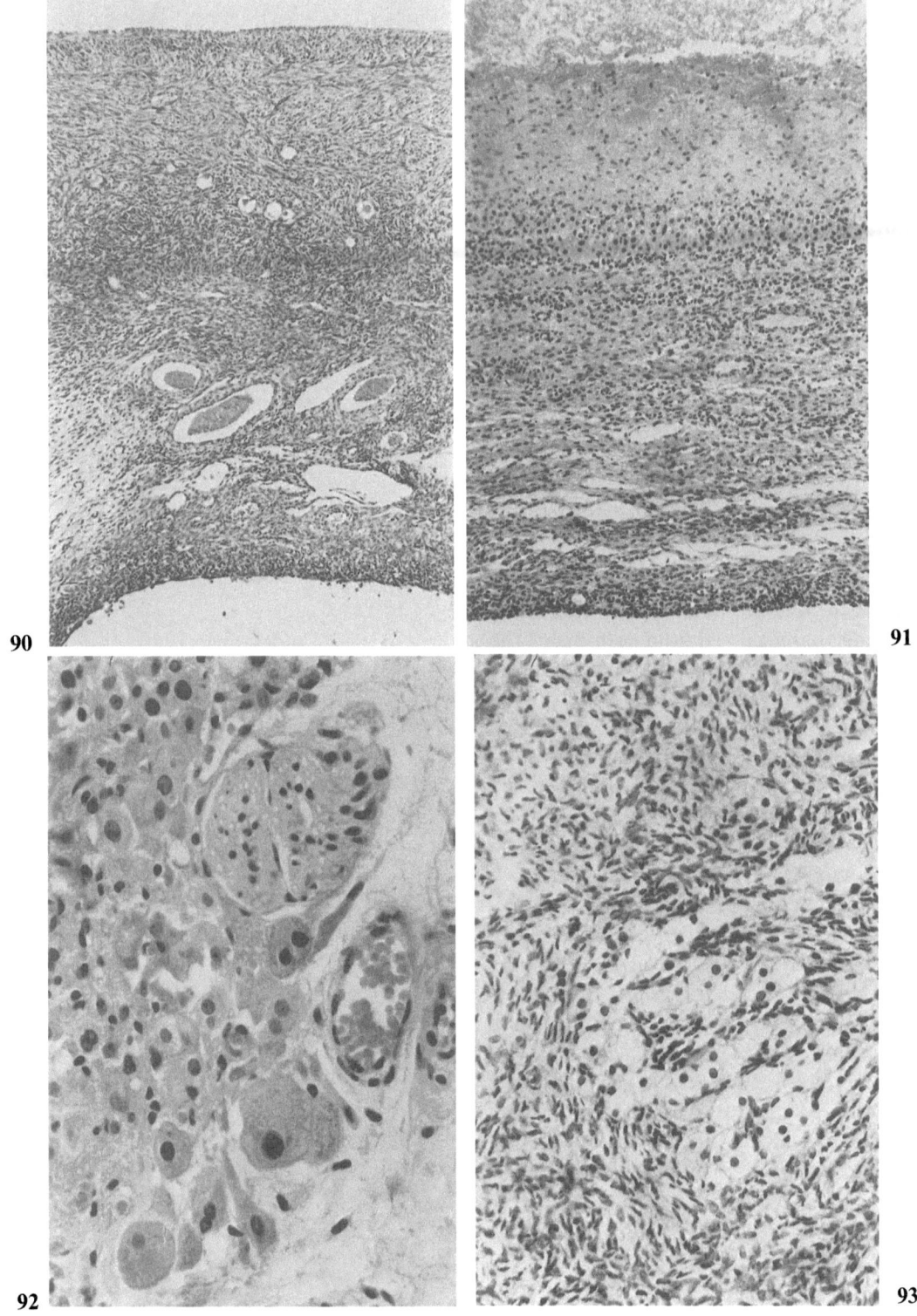

90

91

92

93

Fig. 94 A–D. Serous tumors of the ovary (FIGO I). The cystic serous tumors contain most commonly serous fluid, but in some instances the content may be thick and mucinous, especially in proliferating tumors.

A Serous cystadenoma (FIGO I a). Uni- or multilocular cystic tumor lined with a single layer of regular cuboidal cells, which may be ciliated. × 1050

B Proliferating serous cystadenoma (FIGO I b) (Serous tumor of borderline malignancy, serous carcinoma of low malignant potential). The serous epithelium proliferates and forms numerous small papillae without stroma. The nuclei are irregularly enlarged, some mitoses may be present but there is an absence of stromal invasion. Such tumors often have numerous psammoma bodies, microcalcifications with a concentric arrangement. × 335

C Serous cystadenocarcinoma (FIGO I c). Well-differentiated area of a serous cystadenocarcinoma with multiple invading papillary structures. × 135

D Dedifferentiated area of the same carcinoma as illustrated in C. There are solid masses of tumor cells with pleomorphic hyperchromatic nuclei and numerous mitotic figures. If the whole tumor presented this aspect, it would have to be classified as an undifferentiated carcinoma (FIGO V). × 335

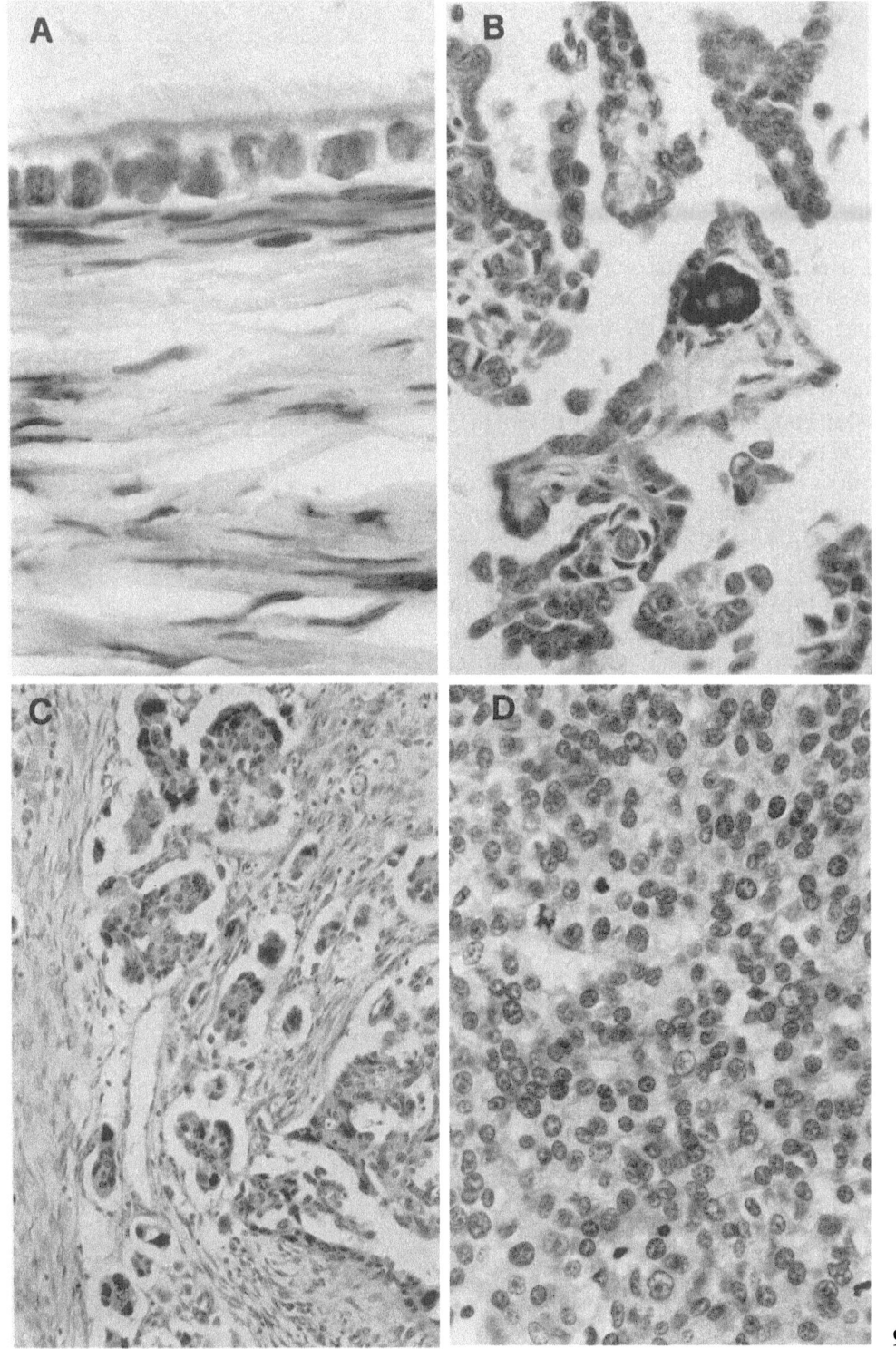

Fig. 95 A–C. Mucinous tumors of the ovary (FIGO II). Intraoperative rupture of a mucinous tumor may lead to the development of pseudomyxoma peritonei. The content of the cysts is usually strongly mucinous and thick, but it also may be thin and watery.

A Mucinous cystadenoma (FIGO IIa). Uni- or multilocular cystic tumor lined with a single layer of regular, tall-columnar, mucus-containing cells. The nuclei are basally located, the cytoplasm contains abundant mucin, which is alcian-blue-positive. ×335

B Proliferative mucinous cystadenoma (FIGO IIb) (mucinous tumor of borderline malignancy, mucinous carcinoma of low malignant potential). The lining epithelium proliferates forming papillary and glandlike structures. The nuclei are irregular, mitoses are present, and mucin production is often decreased. There is an absence of invasive growth. According to some authors, if the atypical epithelial lining is more than three cell layers thick, the diagnosis of carcinoma must be made even when stromal invasion is absent. ×210

C Mucinous cystadenocarcinoma (FIGO IIc). The dedifferentiation of the tumor tissue is evident. The mucin production is considerably decreased. The tumor cells are arranged in glandular and solid patterns. There is definite invasive growth. ×135

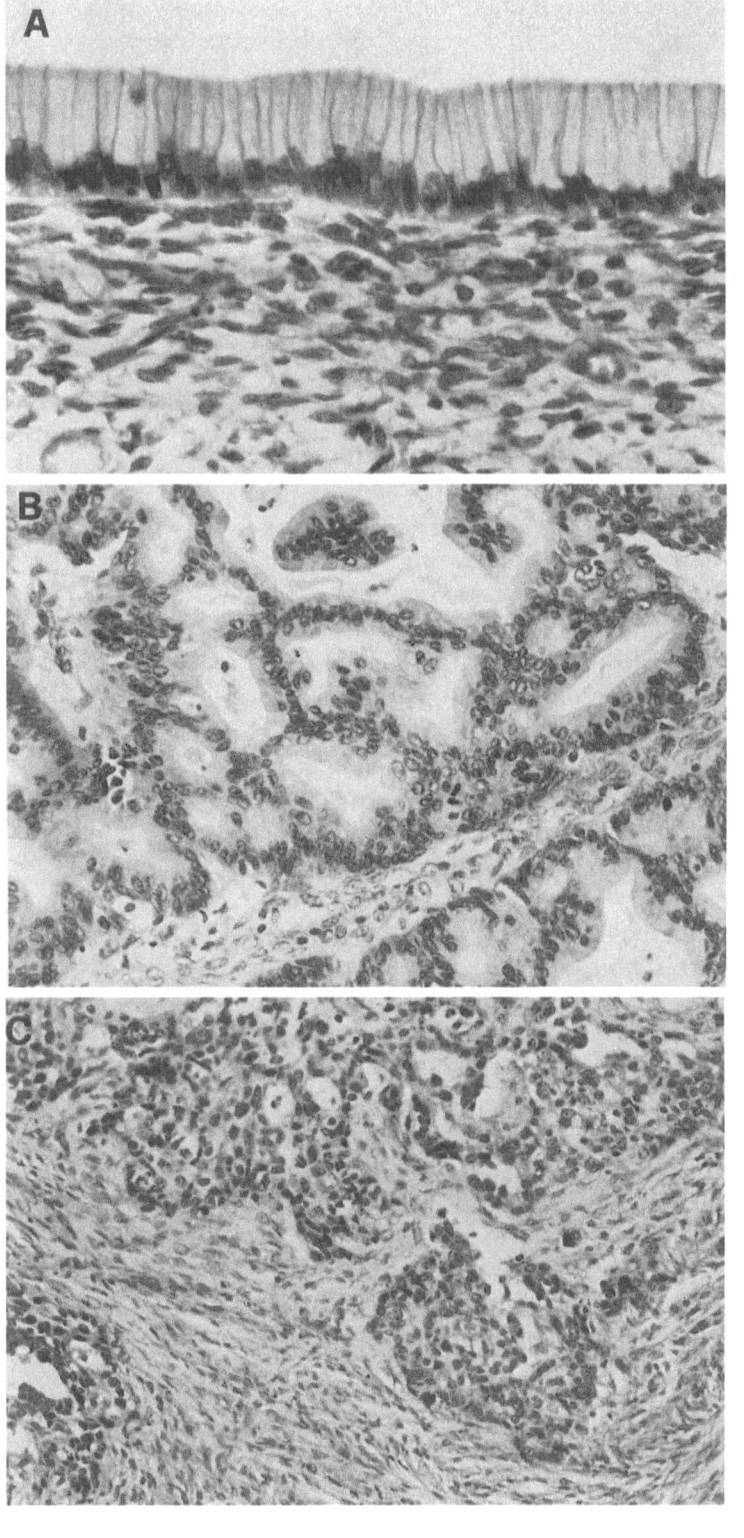

95

Fig. 96 A–C. Endometrioid tumors of the ovary (FIGO III).

A Ovarian endometriosis (FIGO III a). This condition presents most commonly as cysts which are filled with dark brown blood (chocolate cysts). They are lined with endometrium (glands and stroma) and reveal evidence of cyclic haemorrhage. (200×)

Total atrophy of the lining endometrium may occur, thus obliterating the nature of the cyst. Endometriosis may also develop on the ovarian surface, the cyclic bleeding in the peritoneal cavity causing lower abdominal pain.

B Proliferative endometriosis (FIGO III b). In this rare condition, histological changes are similar to glandular or atypical adenomatous hyperplasia of the endometrium. The epithelium may be multilayered, the nuclei are enlarged and hyperchromatic with prominent nucleoli. Mitoses are present but there is no stromal invasion. (160×)

C Endometrioid carcinoma (FIGO III c). These carcinomas are histologically identical to those of the endometrium. Papillary carcinomas and adenocarcinomas with squamous differentiation may also occur. (160×)

The finding of a concomitant endometrial carcinoma is relatively frequent. In such cases it is often impossible to decide whether these ovarian and endometrial cancers are independant primaries or metastatic from each other.

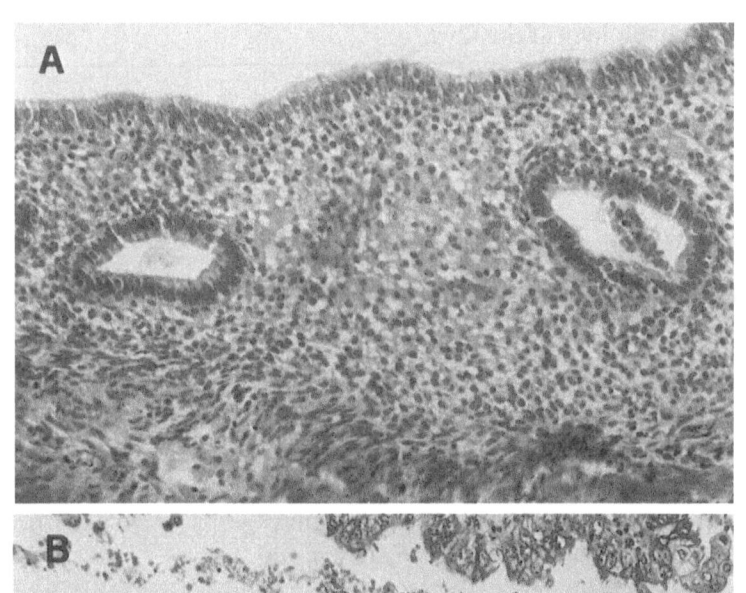

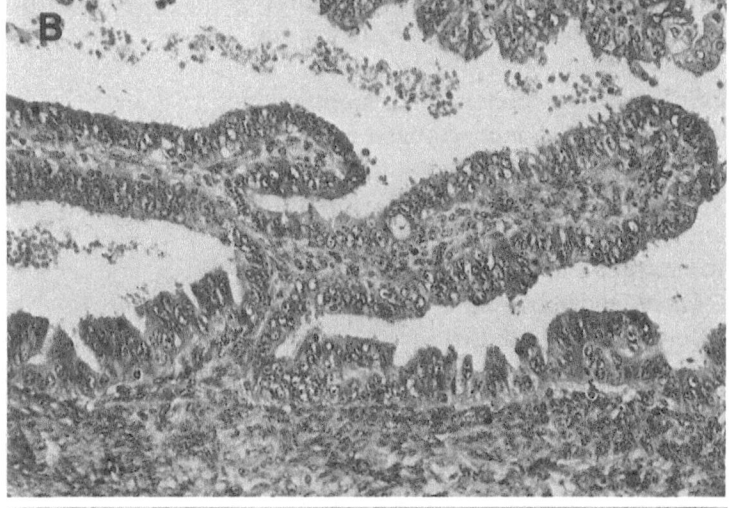

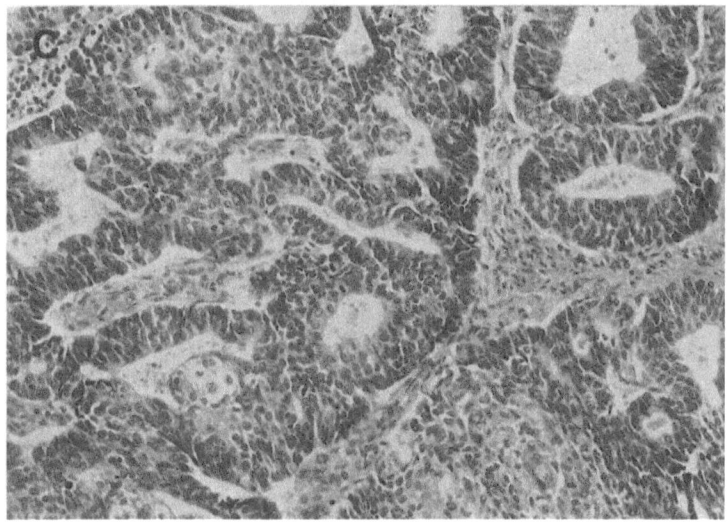

96

79

Fig. 97 A–C. Clear-cell carcinoma of the ovary (FIGO IV c). These tumors constitute about 8% of all primary ovarian carcinomas. They are partly solid adenocarcinomas that are histologically very similar to renal carcinoma. Important differences exist however between both malignancies at the ultrastructural level. Clear-cell carcinomas may occasionally be associated with hypercalcemia.

A Solid pattern of clear-cell carcinoma. The tumor cells are arranged in solid nests and cords. They have distinct cell borders and abundant clear cytoplasm, which contains glycogen. The nuclei are pleomorphic and hyperchromatic. ×210

B Tubuloglandular pattern of clear-cell carcinoma. The tubuloglandular formations are lined with clear cells and with so-called hobnail cells. Small papillary projections centered on a blood capillary are commonly seen. ×135
Differential diagnosis: endodermal sinus tumor!

C Typical hobnail cells. This gland is lined with hobnail-shaped cells which have a nucleus in the apical location and a fine-granular eosinophilic or clear cytoplasm. ×210

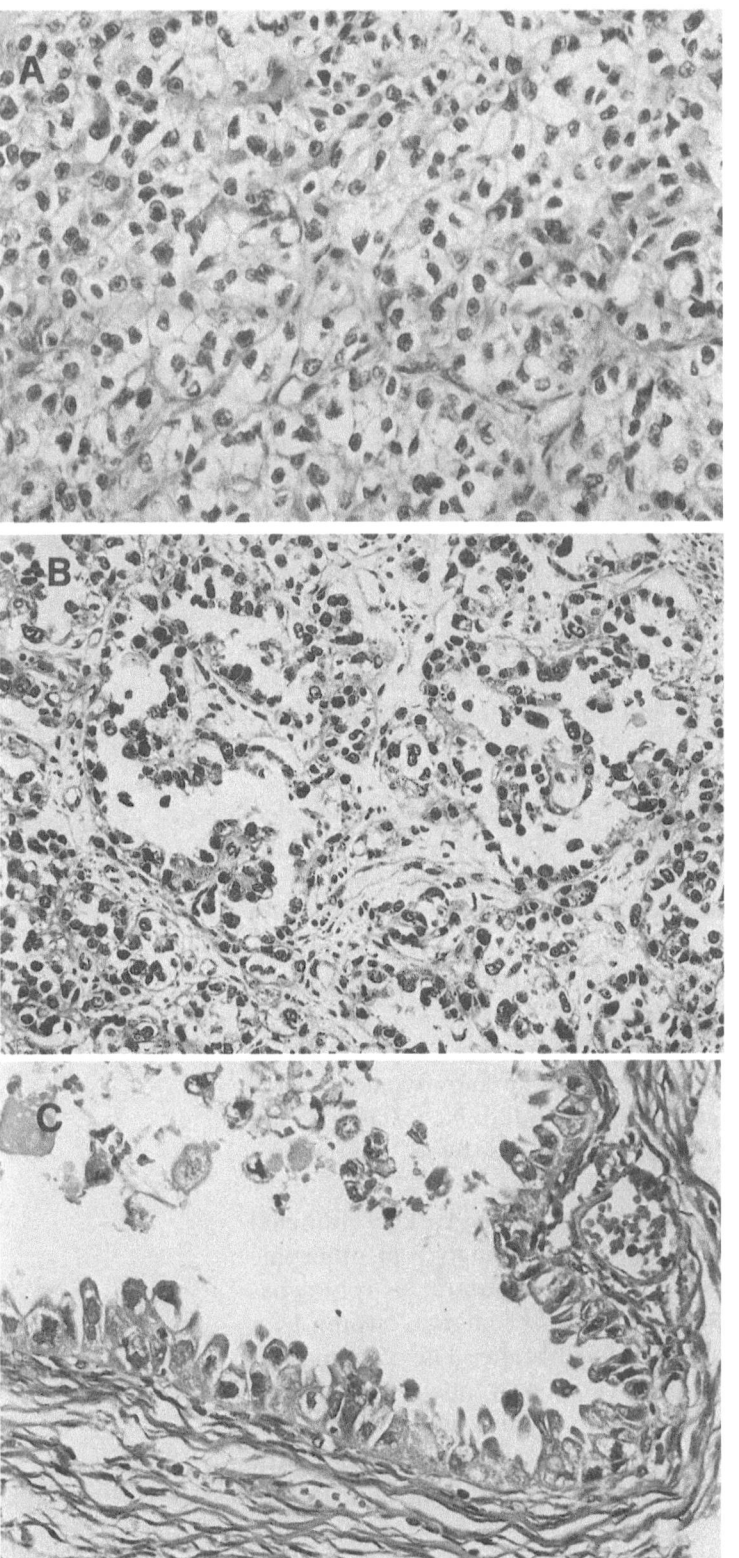

Fig. 98. Undifferentiated ovarian carcinoma (FIGO V). The tumor cells are arranged in solid masses and show no differentiation. The nuclei are strongly pleomorphic and mitotic figures are numerous. ×210

A careful search for better differentiated areas may permit such ovarian malignant tumors to be classified according to the categories illustrated above. In all ovarian tumors, extensive sampling is necessary as the grade of differentiation of the tumor may show considerable variation from one area to another.

Fig. 99 A, B. Malignant mixed mesodermal tumors of the ovary. These are rare ovarian primary tumors. They have been occasionally shown to develop in ovarian endometriosis. Histologically, they are identical to their endometrial counterparts.
A Homologous malignant mixed mesodermal tumor (carcinosarcoma). Some carcinomatous glandular formations are present, surrounded by a sarcomatous stroma. ×85.
B Same tumor as in A: The epithelial cells display strongly pleomorphic nuclei. The epithelium is sharply separated from the sarcomatous stroma by a basement membrane. The sarcomatous elements are polygonal to spindle-shaped with highly pleomorphic and hyperchromatic nuclei. Partly atypical mitoses are present. ×335

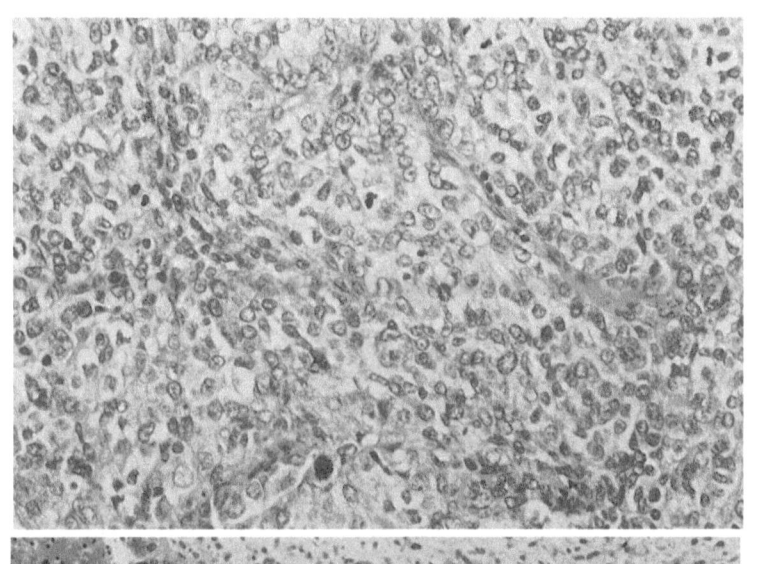

98

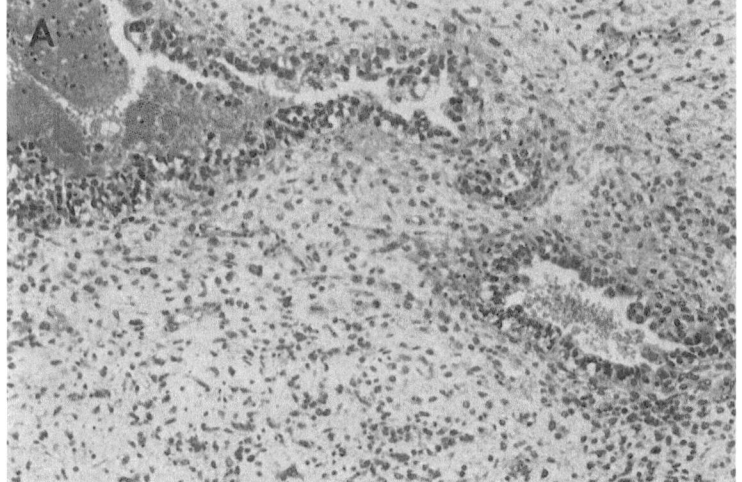

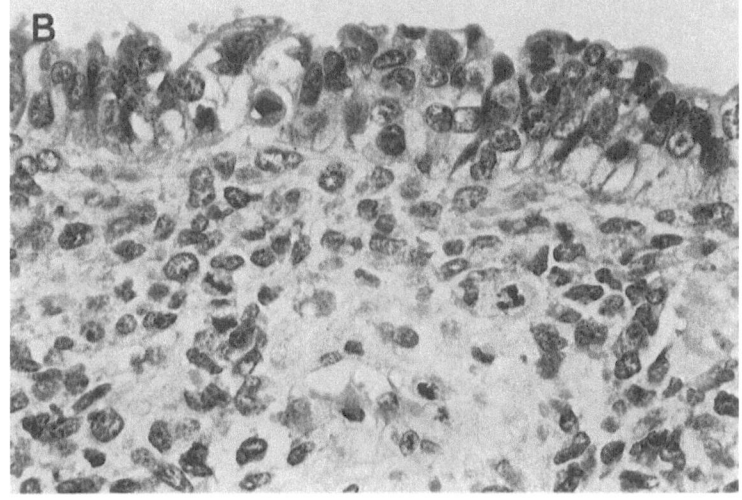

99

Sex Cord Stromal Tumors

Granulosa-Theca Cell Tumors

These neoplasms mostly show endocrine activity and produce estrogens; rarely, they may secrete testosterone. Many tumors contain both theca and granulosa cells. Pure thecomas are benign tumors as a rule. Conversely, 20%–40% of granulosa cell tumors behave in a malignant fashion, and tumor relapse and metastases may develop up to 15 years after removal of the primary tumor. The malignant potential of these tumors is very difficult to assess histologically but mitotic activity may provide some indication.

Fig. 100. Fibrothecoma. The tumor tissue is composed of more or less densely packed spindle-shaped cells. Many cells are fibrocytes or fibroblastlike cells. Scant collagen fibers and some intercellular substance are present between the cells. The theca cells are individually surrounded by reticulin fibers. × 85

Fig. 101. Granulosa cell tumor. The neoplastic granulosa cells contain typical oval coffee-bean nuclei with a longitudinal groove. They are arranged here in the typical microfollicular pattern, forming numerous Call-Exner bodies. In the center of these structures, there is some PAS-positive material and cellular detritus. These glandlike formations are not surrounded by reticulin fibers. × 335

Fig. 102. Granulosa cell tumor (watered silk pattern). The tumor cells are arranged in narrow bands, which are separated by thecal elements, scant connective tissue, and blood vessels. × 335

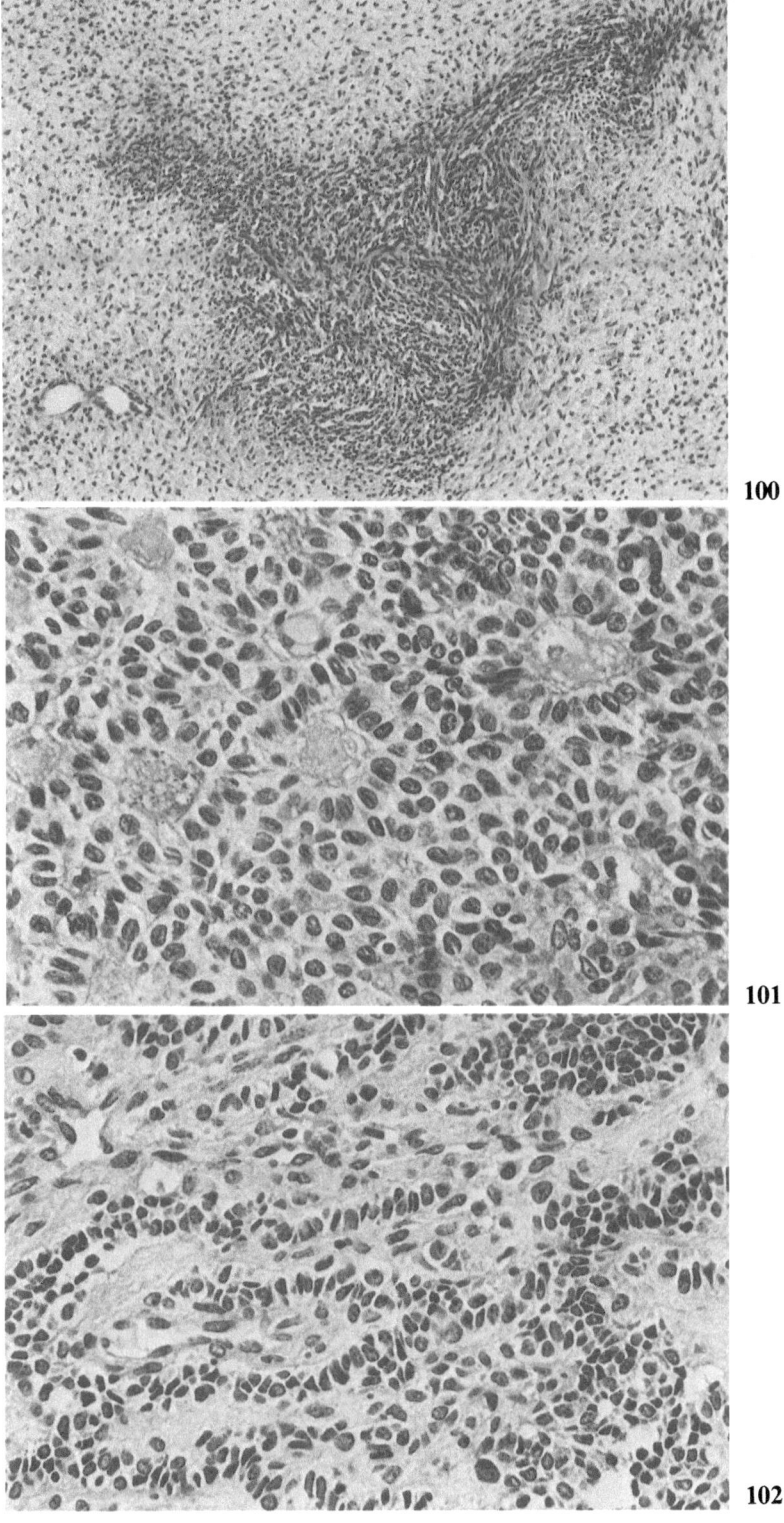

100

101

102

Fig. 103. Granulosa cell tumor (trabecular pattern). The tumor cells are arranged in broad bands separated by thecal elements and connective tissue. ×335

Fig. 104. Granulosa cell tumor (diffuse pattern). The tumor tissue consists of solid growing masses of granulosa cells. A rosettelike arrangement of the tumor cells may occasionally be recognizable. ×335

Fig. 105. Granulosa cell tumor (pseudosarcomatous pattern). The tumor cells are spindle-shaped with elongated nuclei and are arranged in interlacing bundles. A few cells, possibly thecal elements, are luteinized. ×335

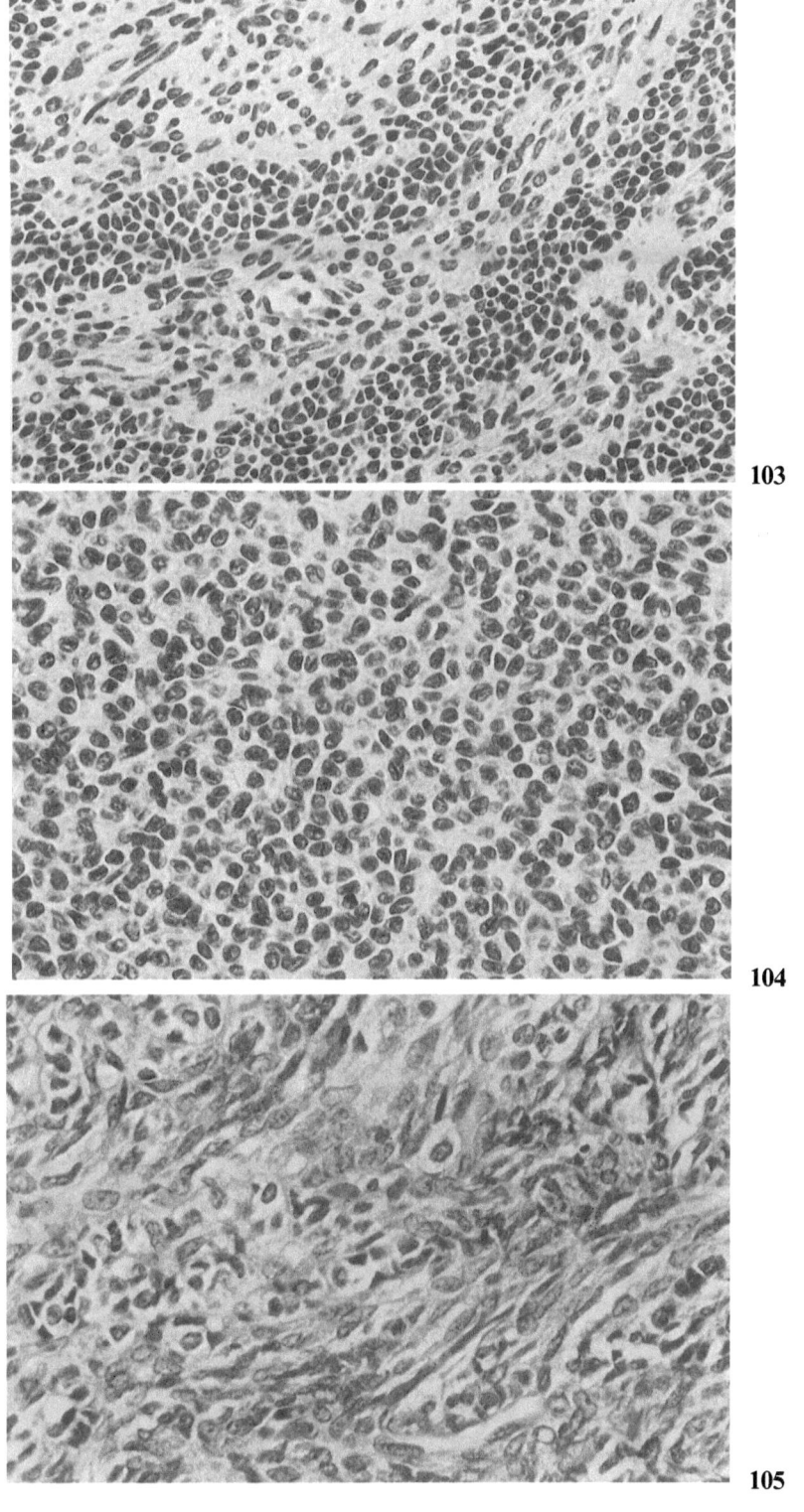

103

104

105

87

Sertoli-Leydig cell tumors

These neoplasms are also called androblastomas. They are most often benign and show endocrine activity. They commonly produce testosterone but some tumors have been shown to be estrogenic.

Fig. 106. Well-differentiated Sertoli-Leydig cell tumor. The Sertoli-like cells are arranged in regular tubules which are separated by small nests of Leydig cells. × 335

Fig. 107. Moderately differentiated Sertoli-Leydig cell tumor. Sertoli cells are arranged in solid nests and cords. Leydig cells contain typical crystals of Reinke. × 840

Fig. 108. Poorly differentiated Sertoli-Leydig cell tumor. The Sertoli-like cells, quite reminiscent of granulosa cells are arranged in large solid sheets. Tubular structures are only rarely found. × 335

Fig. 109. Hilus (Leydig) cell tumor. This tumor is rare, most often benign, and consists solely of hilus cells. It is quite similar to luteinized thecoma and identification of crystals of Reinke is necessary to confirm the diagnosis. The tumor cells have indistinct cell borders, the cytoplasm is abundant and eosinophilic, the nuclei are round with a solitary eccentric nucleolus. × 335

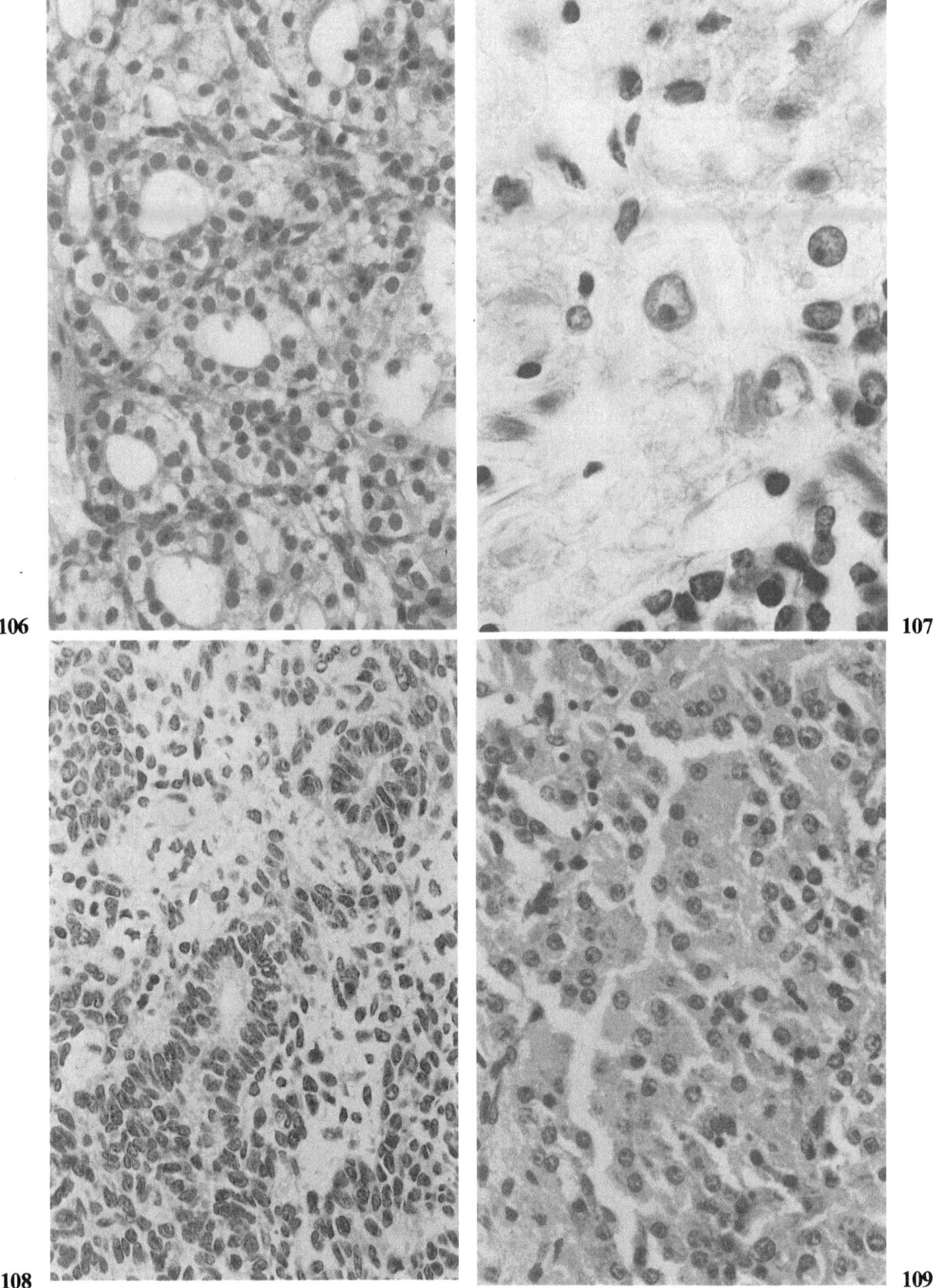

106

107

108

109

Germ Cell Tumors of the Ovary

Fig. 110A–C. Dysgerminoma. This germ cell tumor is highly radiosensitive and is morphologically identical with seminoma of the testis. The typical tumor cells are arranged in nests and cords separated by more or less connective tissue. The neoplastic germ cell is round, oval, or polygonal; the cytoplasm is abundant and pale eosinophilic. The nuclei are enlarged, round, and hyperchromatic. Mitoses are present in moderate number. The intervening connective tissue is more or less infiltrated by lymphocytes. The intensity of lymphocytic infiltration seems to be of some prognostic significance. Occasionally, a granulomatous reaction and giant cells are present.

A Typical dysgerminoma with scant intervening connective tissue and moderate lymphocytic infiltration. ×210

B Typical tumor cells with indistinct cell borders, almost clear cytoplasm, and enlarged and hyperchromatic nuclei. Some mitoses are present. ×335

C This tumor displays a prominent lymphocytic infiltration as well as a focally developed granulomatous reaction with giant cells. ×210

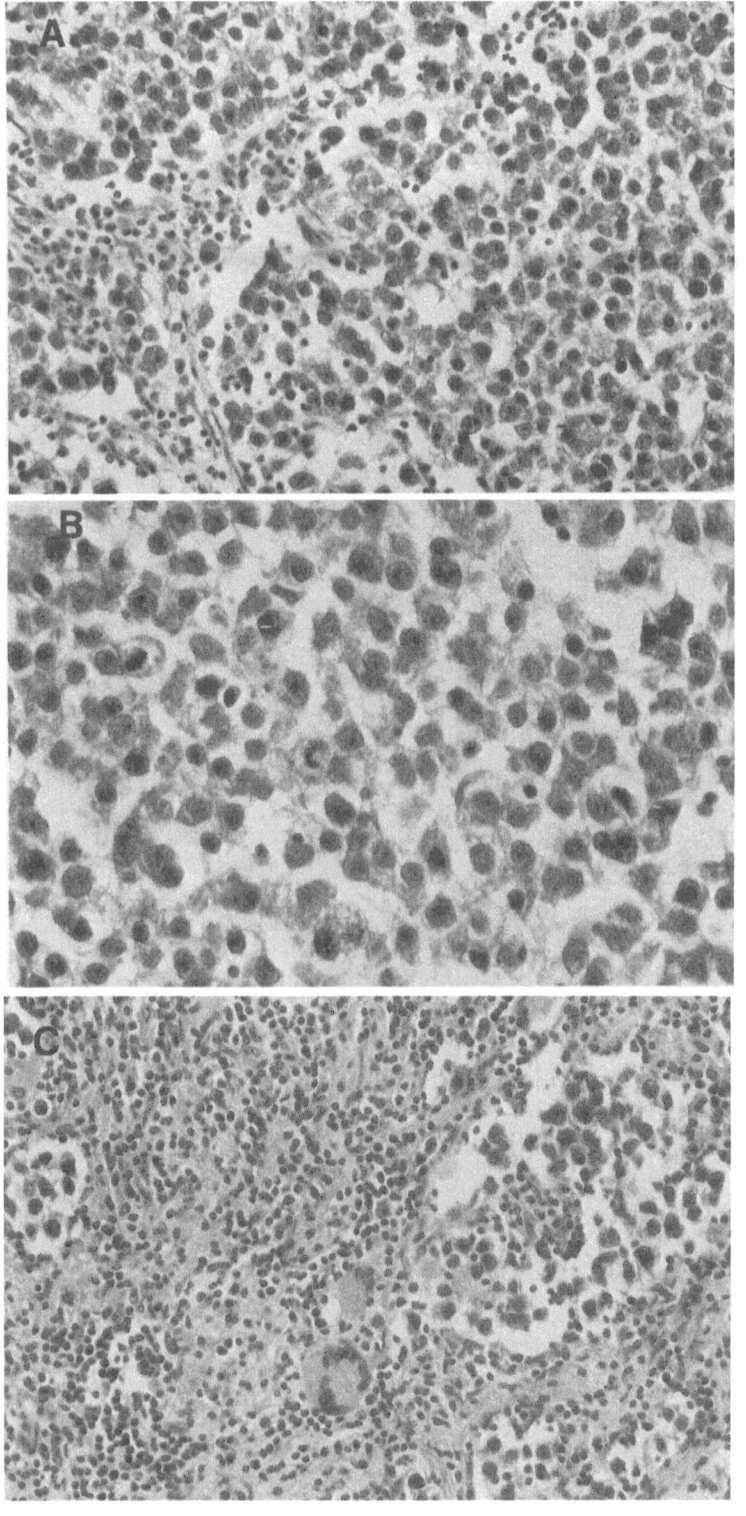

Fig. 111 A–D. Endodermal sinus tumor. This highly malignant tumor is uncommon and occurs mostly in children, adolescents, or young adults. Usually, the tumor cells produce considerable amounts of α-fetoprotein, which may be used as tumor-marker. Histologically, the tumor tissue has an embryonal aspect and consists of solid and small cystic areas. Small papillary formations with a capillary blood vessel in their center (Schiller-Duval bodies) are characteristic of this tumor type. The alveolar, cystic, and tubular structures are lined with cuboidal to flattened cells, which resemble endothelial cells. The solid areas are composed of totally undifferentiated mesoblast, which has an embryonal appearance and may be myxomatous. Most often, some round hyaline bodies or globules are found, which are PAS-positive and contain α-fetoprotein. These hyaline bodies are intra- and extracellular.

A Typical perivascular papillary formation in a sinusoid space (Schiller-Duval body). ×210

B Solid and small cystic pattern with some perivascular glomeruluslike structures. ×210

C Solid undifferentiated pattern with numerous hyaline bodies. ×335

D Small cystic areas reminiscent of the so-called polyvesicular vitelline pattern. ×135

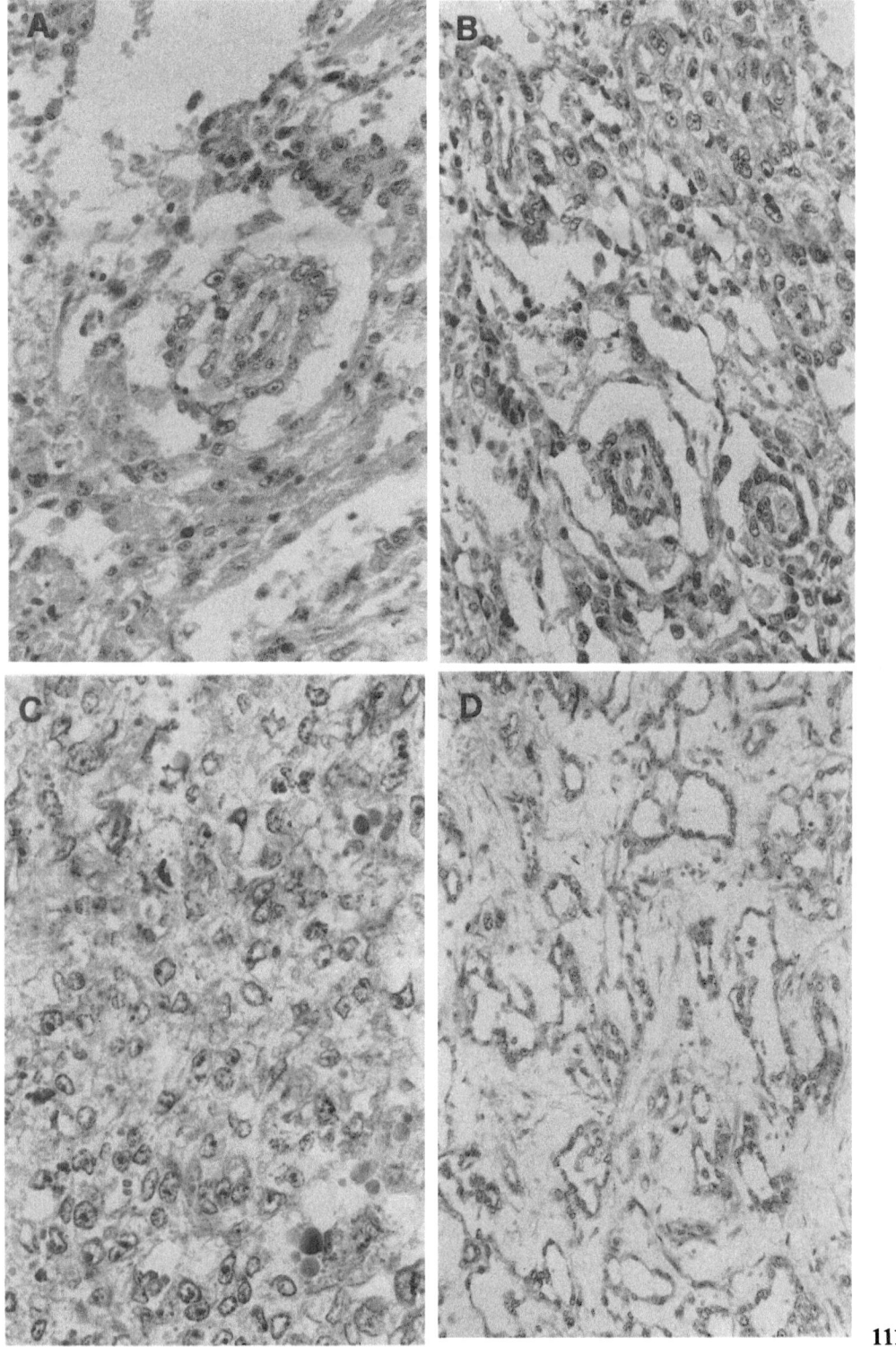

111

Mature Ovarian Teratomas

These benign tumors, which are practically always cystic, contain mostly ectodermal derivatives. The cystic cavities are filled with fatty material, which may be fluid, and hair. In the solid areas, practically every kind of mature adult tissue may be represented. Special types of teratomas, the monodermal developed tumors, are the struma ovarii, the primary ovarian carcinoid, and the strumal carcinoid. Malignant transformation in mature teratomas is a rare event. In such instances, the malignant component is most commonly a squamous cell carcinoma but other carcinomas and some sarcomas have also been reported. Such a malignant transformation occurs predominantly in elderly women.

Fig. 112. Mature cystic teratoma. The lining of the cyst is composed of skin with its various appendages. ×25

Fig. 113. Mature cystic teratoma. Cartilage and bone are frequent mesodermal derivatives found in these tumors. Completely developed teeth are also common. ×53

Fig. 114. Mature cystic teratoma. Mature brain tissue with ganglion cells. ×210

Fig. 115. Struma ovarii. In this case, the whole tumor is composed of thyroid tissue. In some rare instances, malignant changes have been observed. ×210

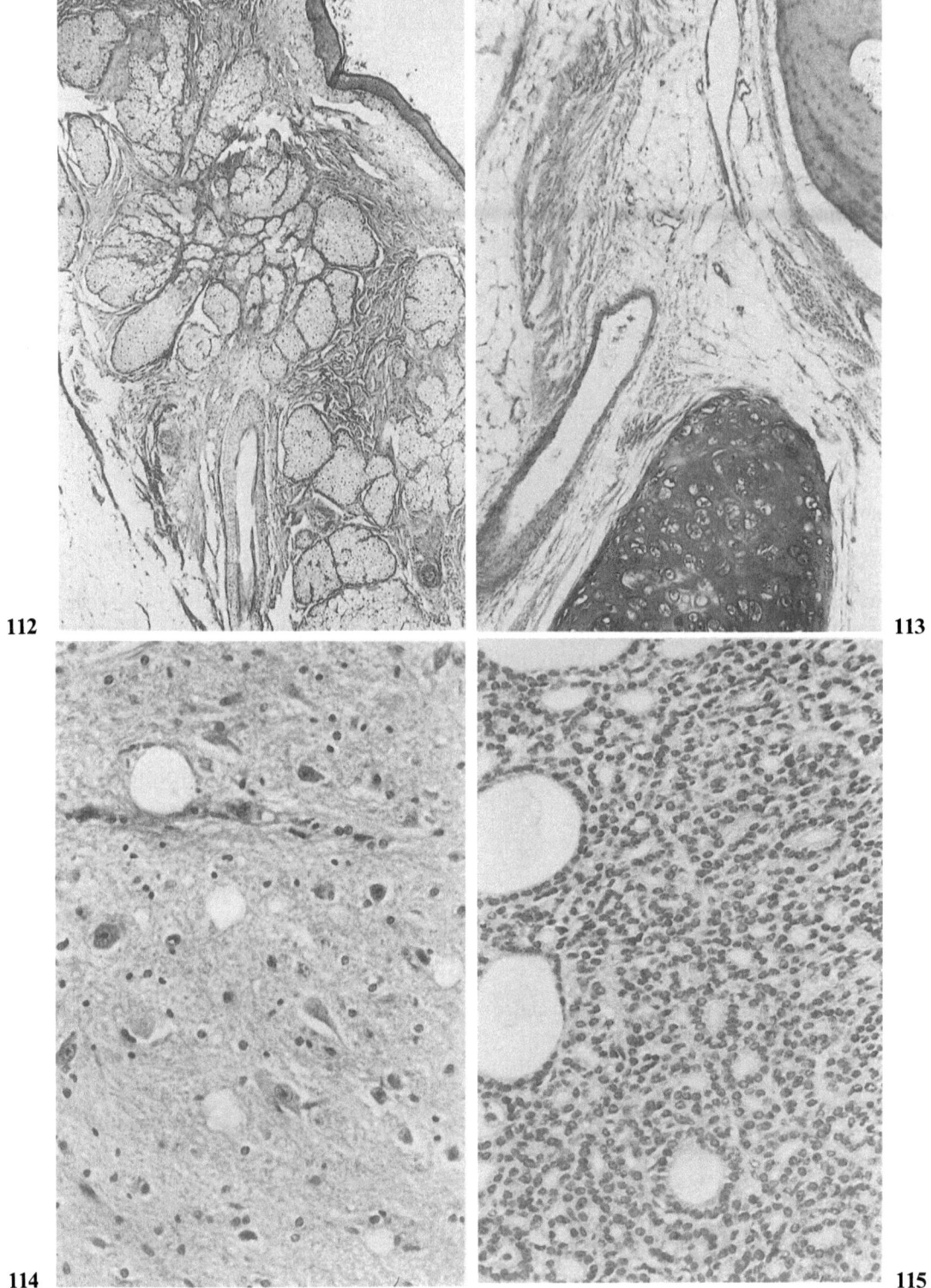

112

113

114

115

Fig. 116. Primary ovarian carcinoid. Morphologically, this type of tumor is identical with the carcinoids in other locations. The primary ovarian tumors behave in a malignant fashion, they may metastasize and cause the development of a carcinoid syndrome. × 110

Immature Ovarian Teratomas

These malignant tumors are rare and occur mostly in children and adolescents. Immature teratomas are usually solid. Histologically, they are most commonly composed of a variety of immature and mature tissues derived from all three germ cell layers. Ectoderm is usually represented by nervous tissue, glia, ganglion cells, neuroblastic tissue, and occular structures. The most common mesodermal derivates are cartilage, bone, smooth muscle, and undifferentiated embryonic mesenchyme. Endodermal derivates are usually present as tubules lined with gastrointestinal or bronchial epithelium.

Fig. 117. Immature bone tissue and glandular structures are present in an undifferentiated mesenchyme. × 85

Fig. 118. Immature cartilage and neuroepithelial elements. × 67

Fig. 119. Neuroepithelial rosette surrounded by glial elements. × 210

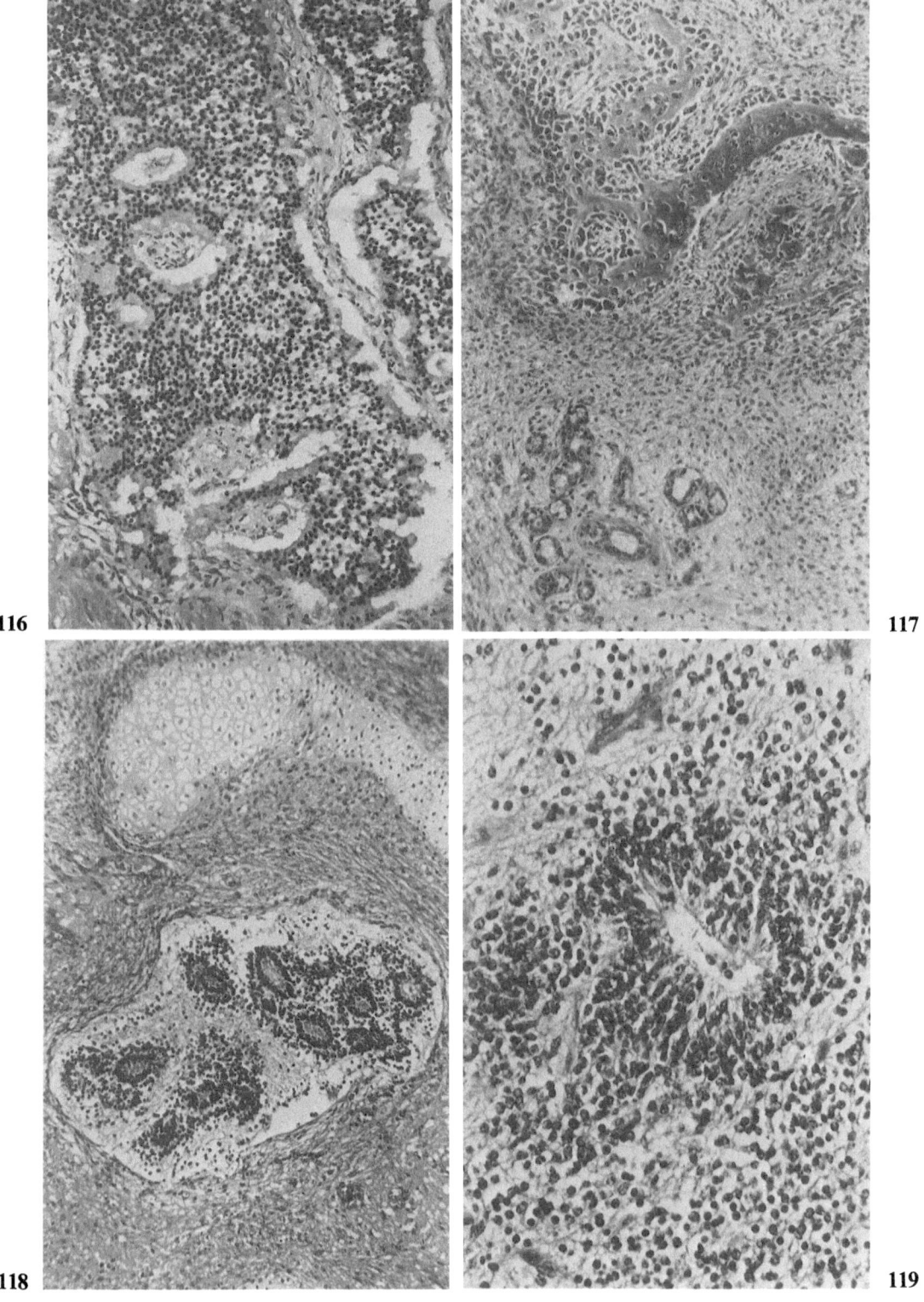

116

117

118

119

The Brenner Tumor

This tumor of unclear histogenesis is almost invariably benign. Histologically, it is composed of solid islands of urothel-like epithelium surrounded by a tightly packed stroma. The epithelial elements are regular, the nuclei are oval with a longitudinal groove, and the cytoplasm is pale. The larger epithelial islands are often cystic and the innermost cell layer undergoes mucinous metaplasia.

Fig. 120. Typical Brenner tumor. The larger epithelial nest shows cavitation beginning. ×67

Fig. 121. Brenner tumor. Cystic transformation of an epithelial island. The innermost cell layer has undergone mucinous metaplasia. ×210

Cancer Metastatic to the Ovaries

Cancer of the endometrium, breast, and gastrointestinal tract often metastasizes to the ovaries. Other primary malignant tumors with ovarian metastases are rare.

Fig. 122. Breast carcinoma metastatic to the ovary. Numerous groups of tumor cells displaying indian-file and glandular patterns are present in the fibrous ovarian stroma. ×210

Fig. 123. Gastric carcinoma metastatic to the ovary. Typical Krukenberg's tumor. The metastatic tumor cells are distended with PAS-positive mucus and appear as signet-ring cells. ×335

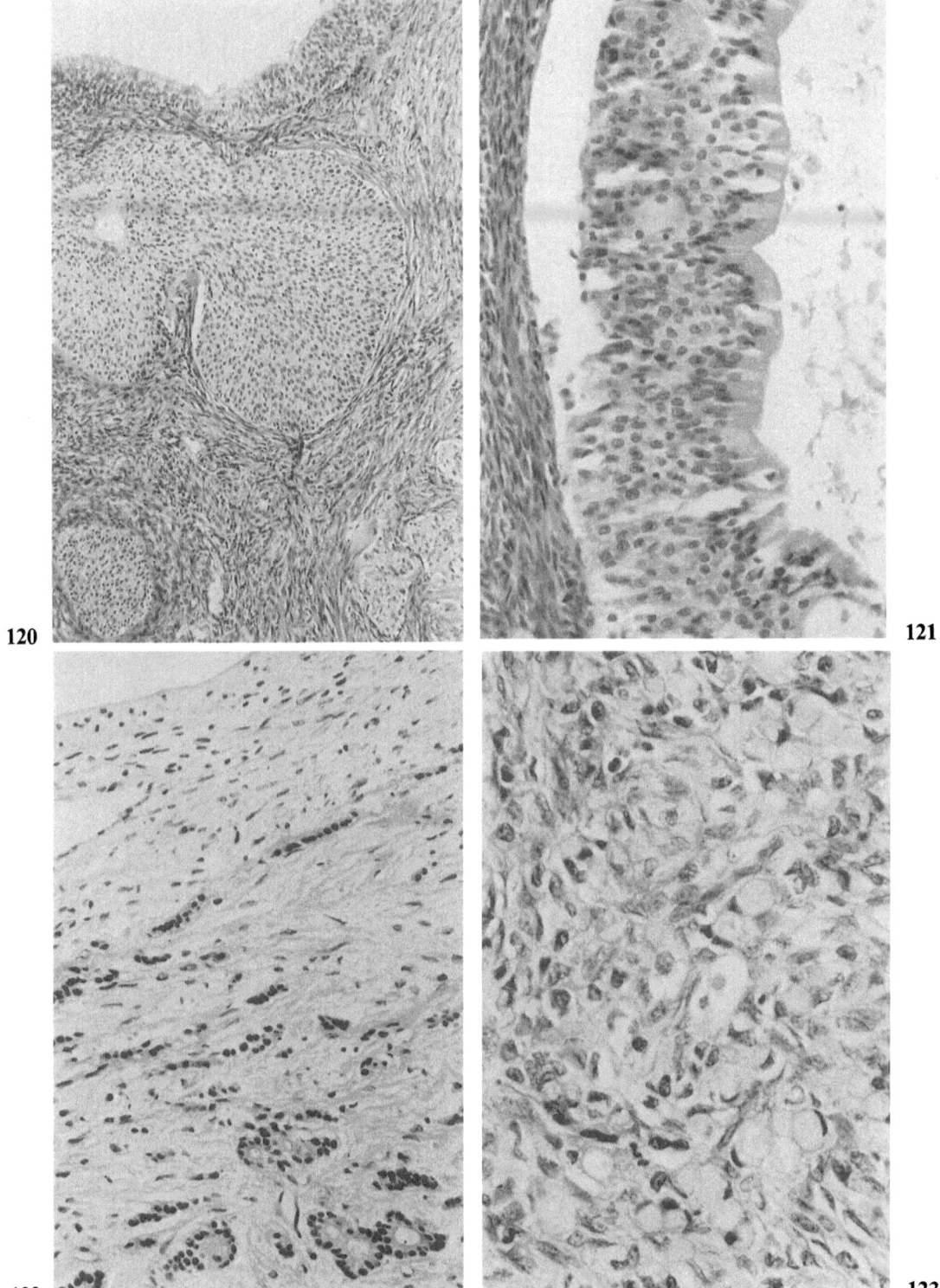

120

121

122

123

99

VIII. Histopathology of Trophoblastic Disease

References

Miller JM Jr, Surwit EA, Hammond CB (1979) Choriocarcinoma following term pregnancy. Obstet Gynecol 53:207–212

Philippe E (1974) Histopathologie placentaire. La maladie trophoblastique. Masson, Paris

Vassilakos P, Riotton G, Kajii T (1977) Hydatidiform mole: two entities. Am J Obstet Gynecol 127:167–170

Hydatidiform Mole

Histologically, this lesion is characterized by hydropic placental villi, which show an absence of fetal vessels and trophoblastic proliferation. The intensity of this trophoblastic proliferation, which provides some information about the malignant potential of the molar tissue, may vary considerably in different areas. Generous sampling of the material is, therefore, recommended. An invasive mole (chorio-adenoma destruens) cannot be diagnosed from curettings alone; the uterus must also be examined. The presence of placental villi in curettings excludes the diagnosis of choriocarcinoma.

A hydatidiform mole must be distinguished from a partial mole in which only some villi show hydropic swelling. In a partial mole, the villi contain fetal vessels and there is an absence of trophoblastic proliferation. A fetus may be present. This condition is most commonly associated with fetal chromosomal abnormalities such as triploidy. Malignant transformation of a partial mole has not yet been recorded.

Fig. 124. Hydatidiform mole. The stroma of the placental villi show considerable hydropic swelling; there is moderate trophoblastic proliferation. ×85

Fig. 125 A, B. Hydatidiform mole. The proliferating cyto- and syncytiotrophoblastic cells show some degree of polymorphism. *A* ×85; *B* ×210

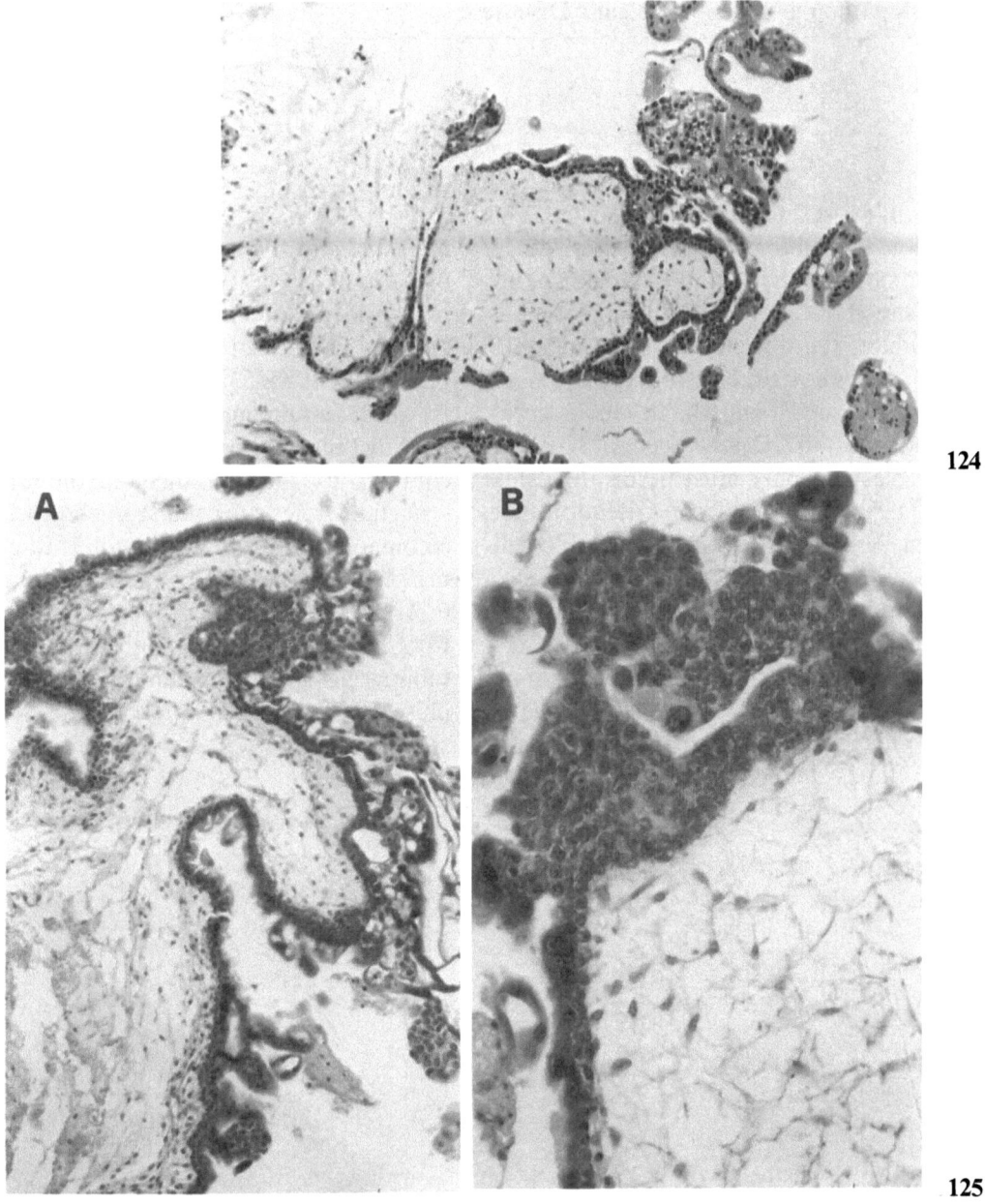

124

A   B

125

Fig. 126 A–C. Choriocarcinoma. This lesion is histologically characterized by pleomorphic cyto- and syncytiotrophoblastic cells, which invade the myometrium in the absence of placental villi. The tumor tissue exhibits extensive necrosis and hemorrhage. Invasion of blood vessels usually occurs. This trophoblastic cancer must be distinguished from the trophoblastic pseudotumor, which is composed of pleomorphic cells resembling trophoblast. The absence of a dimorphic cell population in trophoblastic pseudotumor permits this distinction to be made. Choriocarcinoma can most often be successfully treated by chemotherapy, even if metastasis to the lungs has already occurred. The prognosis is particularly impaired when metastases to the liver and/or brain are present.

A Choriocarcinoma. Malignant invasive growing masses of trophoblast without placental villi. ×53

B Choriocarcinoma. The tumor tissue is invading the myometrium. In contrast to the so-called myometritis syncytialis, the trophoblast in choriocarcinoma invades as large solid tumor masses and the cell population is dimorphic. ×85

C Choriocarcinoma. Both types of tumor cells show considerable pleomorphism. Partly atypical mitoses are present. ×270

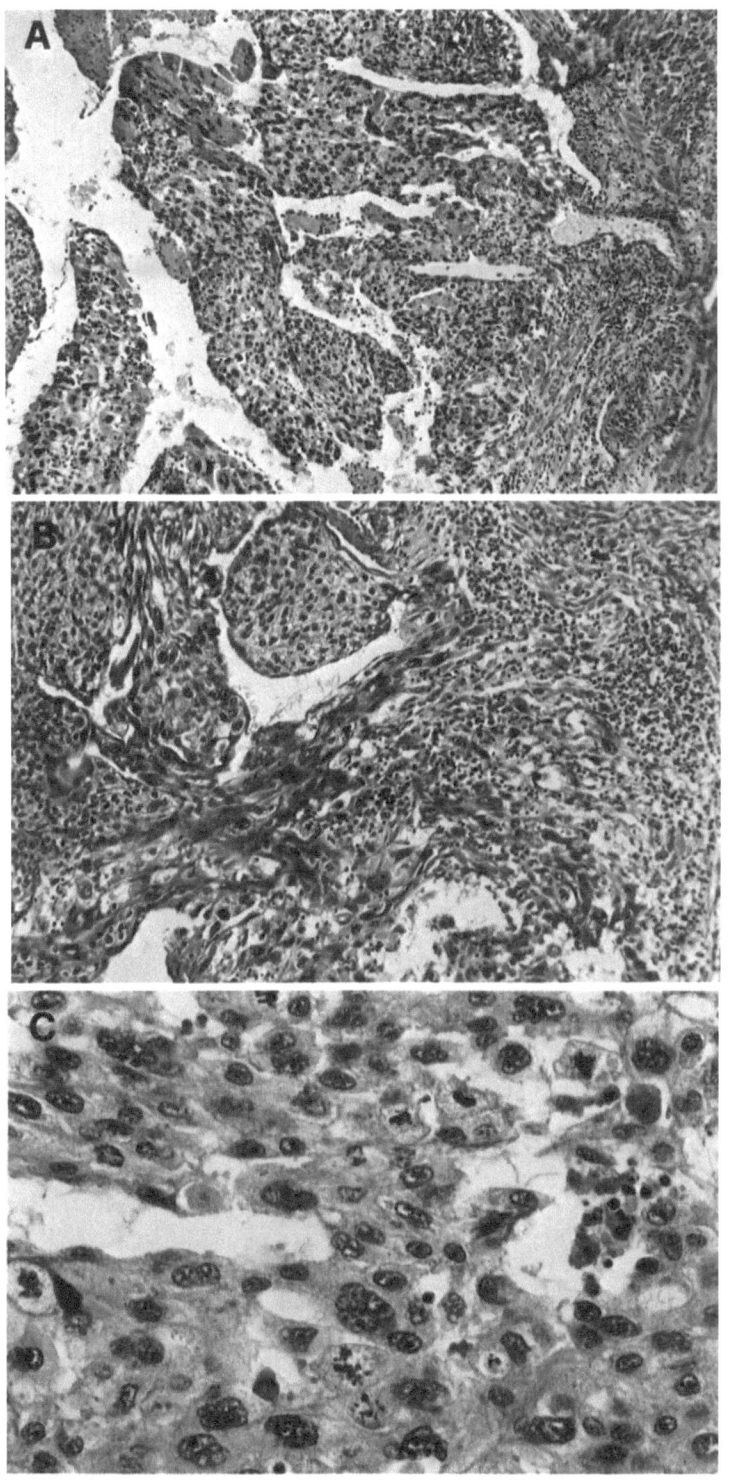

126

IX. Histologic Classification and Staging of Tumors

References

International Federation of Gynecology and Obstetrics (1971) Classification and staging of malignant tumors in the female pelvis. Acta Obstet Gynecol Scand 50: 1–7

Serov SF, Scully RE (1973) Histological typing of ovarian tumors. International histological classification of tumours No. 9. Geneva, World Health Organization

TNM (Tumor, Node, Metastasis) Classification and Clinical Staging of Carcinoma of the Vulva

T. Primary Tumor

T1. Tumor confined to the vulva, 2 cm or less in diameter.

T2. Tumor confined to the vulva, more than 2 cm in diameter.

T3. Tumor of any size with adjacent spread to the urethra and/or vagina and/or perineum and/or anus.

T4. Tumor of any size infiltrating the bladder mucosa and/or the rectal mucosa or both, including the upper part of the urethral mucosa and/or fixed to the bone.

N. Regional Lymph Nodes

N0. No nodes palpable.

N1. Nodes palpable in the groin, not enlarged, mobile (not clinically indicative of neoplasm).

N2. Nodes palpable in the groin, enlarged, firm and mobile (clinically indicative of neoplasm).

N3. Fixed or ulcerated nodes.

M. Distant Metastases

M0. No clinical metastases.

M1a. Palpable deep pelvic lymph nodes.

M1b. Other distant metastases.

Clinical Stage-Groups

Stage I. T1 N0 M0, T1 N1 M0.

Stage II. T2 N0 M0, T2 N1 M0.

Stage III. T3 N0 M0, T3 N1 M0, T3 N2 M0, T1 N2 M0, T2 N2 M0.

Stage IV. T1 N3 M0, T2 N3 M0, T3 N3 M0, T4 N3 M0, T4 N0 M0, T4 N1 M0, T4 N2 M0, and all other conditions containing M1a or M1b.

Clinical Stages in Carcinoma of the Vagina

Stage 0. Carcinoma in situ, intraepithelial carcinoma.

Invasive Carcinoma

Stage I. Carcinoma limited to the vaginal wall.

Stage II. Carcinoma involves the subvaginal tissue but does not extend to the pelvic wall.

Stage III. The carcinoma extends to the pelvic wall.

Stage IV. The carcinoma extends beyond the true pelvis or involves the mucosa of the bladder or rectum. A bullous edema as such does not permit a case to be classed as stage IV.

Clinical Stages in Carcinoma of the Cervix Uteri

Preinvasive Carcinoma

Stage 0. Carcinoma in situ, intraepithelial carcinoma. Cases of stage 0 should not be included in any therapeutic statistics.

Invasive Carcinoma

Stage I. Carcinoma strictly confined to the cervix (extension to the corpus should be disregarded).
I a. The cancer cannot be diagnosed by clinical examination
i. Early stromal invasion.
ii. Occult cancer.
I b. All other cases of stage I.

Stage II. The carcinoma extends beyond the cervix but does not extend to the pelvic wall. The carcinoma involves the vagina, but not its lower third.
II a. No obvious parametrial involvement.

Stage III. The carcinoma extends to the pelvic wall. On rectal examination, there is no cancer-free space between the tumor and the pelvic wall. The tumor involves the lower third of the vagina.
III a. No extension to the pelvic wall.
III b. Extension to the pelvic wall.

Stage IV. The carcinoma extends beyond the true pelvis or involves the mucosa of the bladder or rectum. A bullous edema as such does not permit a case to be classed as stage IV.

Clinical Stages of Endometrial Carcinoma

Preinvasive Carcinoma

Stage 0. Histologic findings indicative of malignancy, carcinoma in situ. Some authors consider atypical adenomatous hyperplasia as carcinoma in situ, others use this term for carcinomas which do not extend into the myometrium.

Invasive carcinoma

Stage I. The carcinoma is confined to the corpus.
Ia. Uterine cavity 8 cm or less.
Ib. Uterine cavity greater than 8 cm.

Stage II. The carcinoma involves the corpus and the cervix.

Stage III. The carcinoma extends beyond the uterus, but not beyond the true pelvis.

Stage IV. The carcinoma extends beyond the true pelvis or obviously involves the mucosa of the bladder or rectum. Bullous edema as such does not permit a case to be classed as stage IV.

The FIGO Cancer Comittee has recommended three grades for the histologic grading of stage I endometrial carcinoma.
G1. Highly differentiated carcinoma.
G2. Differentiated adenocarcinoma with partly solid areas.
G3. Predominantly solid or undifferentiated carcinoma.
The depth of myometrial invasion is of primary importance in the prognosis. Therefore, pathologists should specify whether or not myometrial invasion is present, as well as the proportion of the myometrial thickness affected by the tumor.

FIGO Staging of Ovarian Tumors

Stage I. Growth limited to the ovaries.
Ia. Growth limited to one ovary, no ascites.
  i. No tumor on the external surface, capsule intact.
  ii. Tumor present on the external surface and/or capsule ruptured.
Ib. Growth limited to both ovaries, no ascites.
  i. No tumor on the external surface, capsule intact.
  ii. Tumor on the external surface and/or capsule(s) ruptured.
Ic. Tumor either stage Ia or Ib, but with ascites or tumor cells in peritoneal washings.

Stage II. Growth involving one or both ovaries with pelvic extension.
IIa. Extension and/or metastases to the uterus and/or tubes.
IIb. Extension to other pelvic tissues
IIc. Tumor either stage IIa or IIb, but with ascites or tumor cells in peritoneal washings.

Stage III. Growth involving one or both ovaries with intraperitoneal metastases outside the pelvis and/or positive retroperitoneal nodes. Tumor limited to the true pelvis with histologically proved malignant extension to the small bowel or omentum.

Stage IV. Growth involving one or both ovaries with distant metastases. If pleural effusion is present, only a positive cytology permits a case to be classed as stage IV. Parenchymal liver metastases correspond to stage IV.

Special Category. Unexplored cases thought to be ovarian carcinoma.

Histologic Classification of Ovarian Tumors (WHO 1973)

I. Common "Epithelial" Tumors (see also FIGO Classification)

a. Serous tumors
i. benign: Cystadenoma and papillary cystadenoma, surface papilloma, adenofibroma, and cystadenofibroma.
ii. Of borderline malignancy (carcinomas of low malignant potential): Cystadenoma and papillary cystadenoma, surface papilloma, adenofibroma, and cystadenofibroma.
iii. Malignant: Adenocarcinoma, papillary adenocarcinoma, papillary cystadenocarcinoma, surface papillary carcinoma, malignant adenofibroma, and cystadenofibroma.

b. Mucinous Tumors
i. Benign: Cystadenoma, adenofibroma, and cystadenofibroma.
ii. Of borderline malignancy (carcinomas of low malignant potential): Cystadenoma, adenofibroma, and cystadenofibroma.
iii. Malignant: Adenocarcinoma and cystadenocarcinoma, malignant adenofibroma, and cystadenofibroma.

c. Endometrioid Tumors
i. Benign: Adenoma and cystadenoma, adenofibroma, and cystadenofibroma.
ii. Of borderline malignancy (carcinomas of low malignant potential): Adenoma and cystadenoma, adenofibroma, and cystadenofibroma.
iii. Malignant: Carcinoma, adenocarcinoma, adenoacanthoma, adenosquamous carcinoma, malignant adenofibroma, and cystadenofibroma. Endometrioid stromal sarcoma, mesodermal (Müllerian) adenosarcoma, mesodermal (Müllerian) mixed tumors, homologous and heterologous.

d. Clear-Cell (Mesonephroid) Tumors
i. Benign: Adenofibroma.
ii. Of borderline malignancy (carcinomas of low malignant potential).
iii. Malignant: Carcinoma and adenocarcinoma.

e. Brenner Tumors
i. Benign.
ii. Of borderline malignancy (proliferating).
iii. Malignant.

f. Mixed Epithelial Tumors

i. Benign.
ii. Of borderline malignancy.
iii. Malignant.

g. Undifferentiated Carcinoma

h. Unclassified Epithelial tumors

II. Sex-Cord – Stromal Tumors

a. Granulosa-Stromal Cell Tumors

i. Granulosa cell tumor.
ii. Tumors in the thecoma-fibroma group.
   1. Thecoma.
   2. Fibroma.
   3. Unclassified:
Sclerosing stromal tumor.
Others.

b. Sertoli-Leydig Cell Tumors (Androblastomas)

i. Well differentiated
   1. Sertoli cell tumor; tubular androblastoma (tubular adenoma of Pick)
   2. Sertoli cell tumor with lipid storage, tubular androblastoma with lipid storage (folliculoma lipidique)
   3. Sertoli-Leydig cell tumor (tubular adenoma with Leydig cells)
   4. Leydig cell tumor, hilus cell tumor
   5. Stromal Leydig cell tumor
ii. Of intermediate differentiation
iii. Poorly differentiated (sarcomatoid)
iv. With heterologous elements

c. Gynandroblastoma

d. Unclassified

i. Sex cord tumor with annular tubules
ii. Others

III. Lipid (Lipoid) Cell Tumors

IV. Germ Cell Tumors

a. Dysgerminoma
b. Endodermal Sinus Tumor
c. Embryonal carcinoma
d. Polyembryoma
e. Choriocarcinoma
f. Teratomas
   i. Immature
   ii. Mature
      1. Solid
      2. Cystic:
      Dermoid cyst (mature cystic teratoma)
      Dermoid cyst with malignant transformation
   iii. Monodermal and highly specialized
      1. Struma ovarii
      2. Carcinoid
      3. Strumal carcinoid
      4. Others
g. Mixed Forms

V. Mixed Germ Cell and Sex-Cord – Stromal Tumors

a. Gonadoblastoma
   i. Pure
   ii. Mixed with dysgerminoma or other form of germ cell tumor

VI. Soft-Tissue Tumors Not Specific to Ovary

VII. Unclassified Tumors

VIII. Secondary Tumors (Metastatic)

IX. Tumorlike Conditions

a. Pregnancy luteoma
b. Hyperplasia of ovarian stroma and stromal hyperthecosis

c. Massive edema
d. Solitary follicle cyst and corpus luteum cyst
e. Multiple follicle cysts (polycystic ovaries)
f. Multiple luteinized follicle cysts and/or corpora lutea (hyperreactio luteinalis)
g. Endometriosis
h. Surface-epithelial inclusion cysts (germinal inclusion cysts)
i. Simple cysts
j. Inflammatory lesions
k. Paraovarian cysts

FIGO Histologic Classification of Epithelial Ovarian Tumors

I. Serous tumors
a. Serous benign cystadenomas.
b. Serous cystadenomas with proliferating activity of the epithelial cells and nuclear abnormalities but with no infiltrative destructive growth (low potential malignancy).
c. Serous cystadenocarcinomas.

II. Mucinous Tumors
a. Mucinous benign cystadenomas.
b. Mucinous cystadenomas with proliferating activity of the epithelial cells and nuclear abnormalities but with no infiltrative destructive growth (low potential malignancy).
c. Mucinous cystadenocarcinomas.

III. Endometrioid Tumors (similar to adenocarcinomas in the endometrium)
a. Endometrioid benign cysts.
b. Endometrioid tumors with proliferating activity of the epithelial cells and nuclear abnormalities but with no infiltrative destructive growth (low potential malignancy).
c. Endometrioid adenocarcinomas.

IV. Mesonephric Tumors
a. Benign mesonephric tumors.
b. Mesonephric tumors with proliferating activity of the epithelial cells and nuclear abnormalities but with no infiltrative destructive growth (low potential malignancy).
c. Mesonephric cystadenocarcinomas.

V. Concomitant Carcinoma, Unclassified Carcinoma
Tumors that cannot be allotted to any of the groups I, II, III, or IV.

X. Index

Pathology of the Female Genital Tract

Editor: **A. Blaustein**

2nd edition. 1982. 1249 figures (39in full color).
XIX, 939 pages. ISBN 3-540-90574-X

Updating a highly acclaimed classic reference, this second
edition augments the scope and contents of its predecessor.
Widerly respected contributing authors have provided addi-
tional comprehensive discussions of topics that have become
increasingly important since the publication of the first edition. The expanded coverage includes: clinical correlations
(summaries of symptoms, treatment, prognosis and diagnostic modalities); laser use and colposcopy; prenatal exposure to diethylstilbestrol (DES); malignant diseases; and all
classes of congenital and acquired conditions seen in
women. High quality micrographs and outstanding illustra-
tions complement the text. No other presentation on this
topic is as comprehensive in breadth and depth, making
Pathology of the Female Genital Tract the most valuable
reference for pathologists, gynecologists and gynecology
residents available today.

Functional Morphologic Changes in Female Sex Organs Induced by Exogenous Hormones

Editor: **G. Dallenbach-Hellweg**

1980. 139 figures, 42 tables. XV, 234 pages.
ISBN 3-540-09885-2

This volume contains studies on the functional and
morphological changes in female sex organs following admi-
nistration of estrogen, of gestagen, and of a combination of
hormones. The studies were conducted by researchers the
world over, allowing observations and results from many different regions to be compared and discussed. They will aid
in the recognition of adverse reactions and in the development of methods to prevent them.

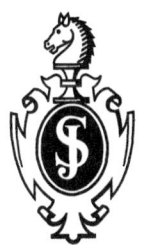

Springer-Verlag
Berlin
Heidelberg
New York
Tokyo

Cervical Cancer

With contributions by numerous experts
Editor: **G. Dallenbach-Hellweg**

1981. 115 figures. VIII, 259 pages
(Current Topics in Pathology, Volume 70)
ISBN 3-540-10941-2

Chronic Pelvic Pain in Woman

Editor: **M. Renaer**

1981. 22 figures, 10 tables. XIII, 197 pages
ISBN 3-540-10608-1

Clinical Trials in 'Early' Breast Cancer

Methodological and Clinical Aspects of Treatment Comparisions
Proceedings of a Symposium, Heidelberg, Germany, 4th to 8th December 1979

Editors: **H. R. Scheuerlen, G. Weckesser, I. Armbruster**

1979. 40 figures, 22 tables. VI, 283 pages
(Lecture Notes in Medical Informatics, Volume 4)
ISBN 3-540-09530-6

Surgery of Female Incontinence

With a Foreword by Sir J. Dewhurst
Editors: **S. L. Stanton, E. A. Tanagho**

1980. 199 figures, 17 tables. XVI, 203 pages
ISBN 3-540-10155-1

Placental Proteins

Editor: **A. Klopper, T. Chard**

1979. 65 figures, 36 tables. X, 171 pages
ISBN 3-540-09406-7

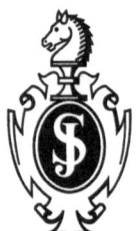

Springer-Verlag
Berlin
Heidelberg
New York
Tokyo